WATER AND SANITATION
Institutional Challenges in India

WATER AND SANITATION

Institutional Challenges in India

Edited by

CHRISTINE SIJBESMA

MEINE PIETER VAN DIJK

IDPAD

MANOHAR

2006

First published 2006

ISBN 81-7304-680-8

Published by
Ajay Kumar Jain *for*
Manohar Publishers & Distributors
4753/23 Ansari Road, Daryaganj
New Delhi 110 002

Printed at
Lordson Publishers Pvt Ltd
Delhi 110 007

Distributed in South Asia by
FOUNDATION BOOKS
4381/4, Ansari Road
Daryaganj, New Delhi 110 002
and its branches at Mumbai, Hyderabad,
Bangalore, Chennai, Kolkata

Contents

CHAPTER 1

Issues in the Water and Sanitation Sector in India

MEINE PIETER VAN DIJK AND CHRISTINE SIJBESMA

INTRODUCTION

India has made noticeable progress towards fulfilling the national and international goals of providing all its citizens with access to improved domestic water supply and sanitation. At the same time, it is experiencing problems in reaching the last of its rural population and urban poor that have not yet been served. An even greater challenge is to sustain the established provisions in such ways that those served now and in future can continue using the improved facilities throughout the years. The growing pressures on water resources and the decentralization of domestic water supply and sanitation to local governments constitute challenges that India is striving to meet in order to provide its entire population with two of the most basic human requirements: a reliable and sufficient supply of safe water for primary needs and decent sanitation.

This book analyses developments in the Indian drinking water supply and sanitation sector in the light of India's recent policy reforms and its growing demand for fresh water in relation to the available water resources. In May 2003, the Indo–Dutch Programme on Alternatives in Development (IDPAD), a programme in which Indian and Dutch development researchers cooperate on topics of mutual interest, supported the organization of a seminar in Delft, the Netherlands. The aim of the seminar was to discuss drinking water and sanitation issues in India, and to relate Indian and Dutch knowledge in this sector. This book is based on that seminar. It gives an overview of the conditions and policies on domestic water supply, sanitation, and water resources management in a wider context. The authors analyse experiences with the implementation of sector reforms in India based on research of government and non-governmental projects and programmes, and make comparisons with integrated water resource management developments in the EU. They show where progress has been made and where constraints and challenges continue. They also identify which further research can help achieve the Millennium Development Goals for the sector: halving, by 2015, the proportions of those who now have no safe water and sanitation and ensuring that the services and programmes become sustainable.

Problems in the water sector in India are extensive, but vary widely from state to state. Besides issues relating to the drinking water and sanitation (for example van Wijk et al., 2002), there are water management issues in particular, concerning the use of scarce resources for agricultural purposes (Put and van Dijk, 1989). The World Bank published a sector review report on urban water supply and sanitation (June 1998) and one on rural water supply and sanitation in India (January 1998; World Bank, 1998a & b). This book discusses research in relation to the rural and peri-urban areas, where the problems of water supply and proper sanitation are most pronounced.

The objective of this chapter is to identify the main water issues in India, which were also discussed during the above-mentioned workshop. The workshop intended to help define research priorities and to formulate a research agenda. Three questions were discussed in the seminar and have prominently been dealt with in the following chapters:

(1) How are institutional reforms created that make it possible to scale up community-managed water services and sanitation programmes under various forms of lowest level management, i.e. different types of partnerships between local government, user organizations and local private sector;
(2) Which demand management and supply efficiency initiatives have brought better water resources management in India;
(3) What is the importance of mobilization of political support and leadership—what makes politicians and administrators become supporters and implementers of new and better sector policies and institutions?

THE DEBATE: WATER MORE THAN H_2O

The book starts and ends with the international context: the changing water resources conditions that make drinking water an increasingly scarce and precious resource. The chapters in Part I sketch the context and give an overview of the current conditions. Besides an overview of the book, Chapter 1 presents the constraints on fresh water that make it crucial that water is managed better all over the world, and also within the drinking water sector. It identifies the problems which face the sector and indicates how the different chapters address these problems. It also states which issues have not been addressed and why this choice has been made.

The seminar started with a debate on the nature of water. Water is a very important issue not only for society, but also for science. Adam Smith had argued that water is decisive, because it determines where people are located, as easy access to drinking water is the foremost factor in deciding ones habitation. During the opening of the seminar Peter Nijkamp, director of NWO, the largest research funding organization in the Netherlands under which the IDPAD programme also falls, argued that water is also extremely important for economists and for economic activities. However, the topic is currently missing on the IDPAD agenda, despite the need for, and knowledge development on, water and sanitation. Water and sanitation are central elements in the human and ecological environment of India and the Netherlands.

Everywhere, people settle near water, for example, near the coasts. It is known that 60 per cent of the world population lives in coastal areas. However, water is also a major source of problems. In the first place, the high urban demand leads to major shortages. Istanbul, for example, will have insufficient water by 2010 or 2015. Water shortages are also a major problem for economic development. In arid lands, unrealistic subsidies for agriculture enhance water shortages by promoting crops which should be cultivated elsewhere. The common agricultural policy of the European Union (EU) leads to overproduction of, for example, olive oil, which could be better produced in arid regions in North Africa.

Nijkamp concluded that water is an economic good and should have a realistic price. However, water is also a complex good. It does not fulfill the normal conditions for an economic good:

(1) The property rights of water are not clearly defined. For example who owns groundwater?
(2) If left to the private sector, the issue changes. It becomes what is the efficiency of a regulatory system complementing private water supply?
(3) The supply of water is often not regular. Who can provide a guarantee that it will be supplied at an affordable price to the poor when it is scarce? Will the private sector do that and at what cost?
(4) Water has different functions: for consumption, industrial use, and agriculture among other things and so prices must also differ by function. However, who can determine these prices?

It was concluded that water has a social and an economic good and its handling is a question for everyone in our societies. A comparison was made with the EU which has the following principles for its water policy:

(1) Full cost recovery (whatever 'full cost' means);
(2) Equity considerations which lead to the adagio that no one can be excluded;
(3) Economic efficiency in supply and delivery is nevertheless important and can be served in certain cases by privatization, for example in the UK;
(4) Solutions should be administratively feasible, which means that there must be no high transaction costs.

Nijkamp drew a number of overall conclusions. First, there is a case for government intervention to ensure good water quality and access for all. In such a system, subsidy is in principle possible, but it need not be on the water itself. Governments can, for example, subsidize low-cost technology to save water. A regulatory system is necessary to avoid the wastages of a monopoly. Providing information to public is desirable to reduce water wastage. The above points should lead to the promotion of the economic use of water. More efficient user technologies should be developed. For example, car cleaning takes only 12 l in Israel, while in the Netherlands, washing may require per car 150–300 l. Finally, Nijkamp concluded that water is an economic *and* social good.

Recent developments in agricultural and domestic water supply in

India are important. Attention needs to be given to the questions of full water charges and differential service levels to sustain an affordable service for all. There are also political problems and issues of governance; service management issues; social issues, especially those of reaching the poor and giving influence and accountability to poor people and women; issues related to the protection of the environment and to treating water as a precious resource; and issues related to which organizations can best support the local governments and user groups to install and maintain services they want and can sustain.

WATER SUPPLY AND SANITATION IN A CHANGING ENVIRONMENT

The reported total water supply and sanitation coverage in India is 88 and 31 per cent respectively. The Sixth Five Year Plan (1980–5) stressed the importance of safe drinking water supply and the importance of improving the quality of the environment (Sunshine, 2002). As part of the Seventh Five Year Plan the GoI launched the Central Rural Sanitation Programme (CRSP) to complement the efforts of the state governments. Chakravarty (1990) gives an overview of programmes involving applications of science and technology to drinking water during the seventh plan. The National Drinking Water Mission (since 1991, the Rajiv Gandhi National Drinking Water Mission) was launched to improve drinking water and related water management. At that time, the objective was to supply 40 litres per capita per day in all of India and 30 litres per capita per day in desert areas for cattle.

The national plan is the instrument to achieve these goals. During the Ninth Five Year Plan (1997–2001), the CRSP was restructured into a demand-driven and people-oriented approach, the so-called Total Sanitation Campaign (TSC, Sunshine, 2002). Rural water supply has also been decentralized, first as a sector reform pilot project and now as part of a national policy and under a large programme, Swajaldhara. To implement the policy and provide safe drinking water to all Indians by March 2004, the Department of Drinking Water Supply was created in 1999 under the Ministry for Rural Development. The drinking water and improved sanitation objectives need to be achieved through the Tenth Five Year Plan (2002–7).

Van Wijk et al. (2002) gives an impression of the country's drinking water and sanitation developments through governmental programmes. The centrally sponsored Minimum Needs Programme and the Accelerated Rural Water Supply Programme have increased access to a safe water source within 1.6 km and in 17 years the percentage of the desired quantity of water per day (40 litres per person) has increased from 31 to 87 per cent in 1997. Almost 95 per cent of the rural population is reported to have at least one source of domestic water that meets the national standards. James et al. (2002) stress the relevance of such a supply for economic development of the poor. When implemented with productive as well as welfare and health objectives, water supply improvement projects can also help create income through micro-enterprises.

NGOs are also active. In the field of sanitation in Gujarat, the Water, Sanitation & Hygiene for All campaign of the WSSCC has, for example, been active and quite successful (WSSCC, 2002) although now concentrating on the needs in relief camps set up to cope with some 1,20,000 citizens displaced by sectarian violence. The essence of this NGO approach is summarized in Box 1.1. Another example of progress comes from Kerala, where an NGO-piloted community management approach to sanitation has mainstreamed to local and state government (van Wijk, 2002).

What explains the progress in the drinking water supply and sanitation sector in India? In the first place it is important that India has a policy in the water sector (Naidu, 2002). The country embarked

Box 1.1: NGO Approach to Hygiene Training

The WASH Campaign is harnessing the skills of local NGOs with health training and education experience to work with camp administrators. The basics do's and don'ts of hygiene behaviour are being combined with efforts to provide mobile toilets. Open defecation is rampant in these locations, few of which have either provision or space for latrine construction. The WASH Campaign has supplied over 90 mobile toilets, through emergency assistance from the Geneva-based WSSCC. Mobile toilets are being used to demonstrate appropriate behaviour in this initial round of hygiene education.

Source: WASH (2002).

on a very bold rural drinking water sector reform programme (see Box 1.2). Initially, this was totally managed by State water agencies and water boards without community participation. The 73rd and 74th constitutional amendments passed in the early 1990s and subsequent state-level legislations and regulations involved the decentralization of 19 functions among which water supply and sanitation were allocated to the local governments. The reforms aim at the empowerment of the village community and its institution as well as emphasizing the inclusion of women, socially disadvantaged and poor sections of the society. NGOs and CBOs are promoted to play a catalytic role to provide capacity support to the people, community and local governments. The reforms are praised because of the community-orientated and participative approach (Jal Manthan, 2002). Some states, such as Kerala, Madhya Pradesh and West Bengal have made substantial advances in decentralization by the re-allocation of development budgets to Panchayats and by starting the process of participatory people and Panchayat-based planning and development. However, the pace of the process is generally considered to be too slow, on account of resistance by vested public and private interests in centralized and subsidized water and sewerage services managed by the State water agencies, and in the face of poorly developed capacities at the Panchayat level.

Box 1.2: Principles to Allocate Water Sector Reform Funds to States

1. The adoption of demand-driven approach and empowerment of villagers;
2. A focus on village-level capacity building;
3. The maintenance of an integrated approach to water supply, sanitation and hygiene promotion;
4. A requirement for partial capital cost recovery and full operations and maintenance financing by users;
5. The promotion of groundwater conservation, rainwater, harvesting.

Secondly, at the state level, different strategies are pursued. An agreement with the national government has been reached to address the priorities listed in Box 1.3. The impression is that state governments have given very low priority to water in general and sanitation specifically.

Box 1.3: Priorities: Central and State Governments in India

1. Supporting effective and inclusive decentralization by empowering local communities in rural areas;
2. Building and implementing consensus on key policy and institutional reforms;
3. Funding investments in rural infrastructure linked to reforms in service delivery;
4. Using NGO and alternative service providers;
5. Promoting cost recovery;
6. Targeting the poorest and must vulnerable groups;
7. Integrating allied interventions for maximum impact.

In the third place, the drinking water and sanitation sector also receives international support by bilateral agencies, for example, grants from Denmark and The Netherlands, and multilateral donors, for example loans from the World Bank. The support is limited in volume, but it has played strategic though not mainstream roles in developing and testing more community-managed approaches with attention to social and gender equity. UN Habitat has started the Water for Asian Cities programme. This stresses pro-poor investment in drinking water supply and sanitation to support millennium development goals. Box 1.4 gives an example of a donor-supported water project.

In the past, the private sector, brought in by UNICEF, has played a crucial role in bringing domestic water services to the rural poor by the licensed production and distribution of a durable and standardized hand pump (Kolsky et al., 1999). More recently, the private sector has shied away from investment in the water sector. This is due to the expectations concerning the returns on these investments. There is a need to base water pricing not only on recovering the operation and maintenance costs, but also to allow recovery of part of the capital cost.

> Ultimately, India will have to go to full water charges according to the Deputy Chairman of the Planning Commission, K.C. Pant (*Businessline*, 11 December 2002). There are, however, also considerable risks that a large-scale introduction of yet other supplies with higher service levels will leave the poor without reliable and nearby water service, unless a system for integrated and equitable management of combined water supplies is developed. (Kolsky et al., 1999)

The question remains under what kind of circumstances drinking

Box 1.4: Donor-supported Water Project

In the Gujarat Rural Water supply Scheme, local women were trained to use water and time gains productively as well as domestically and, with the assistance of SEWA, were able to form cooperative enterprises. In a study of this experience, the gender impacts of both improved water supply and of the income generated through the women's own new enterprises was analysed. In Gujarat, the policy priority of the Netherlands Embassy on gender created the financial room for local actors to come up with innovative projects.

In Kerala, both Danish and Dutch donor insistence on combining water supply with sanitation and citizen participation created space for poor peri-urban groups to exercise control over their basic services. Other than in Gujarat, where the State Water and Sewerage Board continues to control drinking water and sanitation, the shifting political power then could overrule the opposition from the Kerala State Water Authority.

Source: van Wijk et al. (2002)

water supply and sanitation projects can be successful. It should become clear what we know and what still needs to be researched. This book compares the political objectives with research findings on achievements and progress and the identification of subject fields for further study.

The new national policy for water management is presented in Chapter 2 by J.S. Burjia. The policy was revised in 2002 to achieve the desired goals and brings with it a number of new areas for research such as the effects of the bans on water withdrawal and the promotion of economic water use.

Chapters 3 and 4 focus on the situation in drinking water supply and sanitation on the ground. Information on these conditions comes from an analysis of the statistics of the 54th National Sample Survey (NSS) in 1998 and the Census of India of 2001. Traditionally, the public sector in India was assigned a dominant role in planning, development and management of drinking water supply and sanitation projects. In Chapter 3, U. Sankar explores the sustainability of this approach and its alternative of public–private partnerships (PPP). It gives reasons for assigning a dominant role for government in the past, assesses the current status of drinking water supply and sanitation in the rural areas of India in terms of their availability, type of access and quality, and highlights the problems in continuing the centralized supply-driven approach. The author argues in favour of a decentralized demand-driven approach based on PPP.

He identifies the roles for government, private firms and local communities in planning, development and management of drinking water supply and sanitation projects. Sankar also considers the problems of coordination, cost sharing, pricing, access to the poor and economic sustainability. Two examples of PPPs are given to illustrate issues in the design and implementation of PPP.

In Chapter 4, V.R. Reddy and S.M. Dev analyse the general situation in the water and sanitation sector in India. The picture is discomforting and a lot needs to be done to achieve the Millennium Development Goal of halving the number of people not receiving clean drinking water. The World Environmental Conference in Johannesburg in 2002 added the objective of halving the number of people currently not served by improved sanitation, also a very ambitious goal for India, which will not easily be met by 2015, the chosen deadline. New investments need to serve the remaining unserved. Given also the estimated costs of sustaining the already established systems, while these systems are vastly insufficient, alternative delivery systems are presented: partnerships between municipalities or community councils, user associations, and local lenders and firms, alone or in combination with smaller expatriate enterprises and banks.

Chapter 4 also addresses the other side of the coin for supplying more people from the same amount of water. That is better management of the available water, a strategy that has so far been hardly tried and researched. The authors discuss four strategies for water management and based on research elsewhere estimate that savings in water consumption of over 270 per cent are possible in India. Action research can show if and how such savings can be realized, enabling water enterprises to save greatly on new investments to the benefit of upgrading and expanding current services.

WATER MANAGEMENT IN PARTICULAR FOR AGRICULTURAL PURPOSES

Water management has a long tradition in India. In the 1960s the government introduced multi-annual programmes for investments in dams, water reservoirs and irrigation networks. By connecting villages to the electricity grid, farmers were allowed to pump up water for irrigation purposes (Put and van Dijk, 1989). Electric power supply for agriculture is free in certain states and heavily subsidized in others. This has led to excessive exploitation of groundwater. There seems to be a need to do away with subsidies in the power sector, or to introduce an appropriate tariff to act as a disincentive for over-exploitation of groundwater.

Usually, a project approach was chosen to increase the access to irrigation and safe drinking water (for example World Bank, 1998b). Often, support was received from international organizations or local non-governmental organizations (NGO). Put and van Dijk (2000) conclude that in fact the difference between the World Bank and a big local NGO in Andhra Pradesh (AWARE) in their approach to dryland agriculture are not as big as one may have expected.

Recently, the scale for integrated water resources management has been expanded, as illustrated by the Narmada Dam project in Gujarat. This is a major water development scheme to provide drought relief, to help to solve water shortages and contamination by fluorine and saline intrusion close to Gujarat's seashores. This infrastructural project aims to irrigate 19.05 lakh ha. of land in Gujarat and Rajasthan and will provide drinking water to 8,215 villages and 135 cities in Gujarat and 131 villages in Rajasthan. *India Today* (9 September 2002) reports on this project that: 'after years of litigation, the release of Narmada waters to the Sabarmati River brings with it the hope of rich agricultural yields and a better life'.

Whether such progress will happen also depends on the scope and quality of community participation, along with social and gender equality. The importance of community participation in watershed management is recognized. It is necessary from the planning to the management stage and its success is co-decided by the degree to which burdens and benefits are balanced between the genders and the different socio-economic groups. The watershed development approach seems to be more fruitful than trying to revive old tanks in isolation from each other as found for example by the Dahn Foundation, 2002. Without irrigation India would probably suffer from hunger, but irrigation also causes many problems:

(1) Shortages of water;
(2) Lower ground water levels;

(3) Salination of the soil;
(4) Inequitable distribution (see Box 1.5);
(5) Lack of adjustment to other uses of the water such as domestic use, and in the case of dams;
(6) The displacement and deterioration of the livelihood of poor people.

Box 1.5: Local Power System Makes Water Distribution Inequitable

The introduction of sugar cane and rice in the area, crops which both need much water, caused a shortage of water among the farmers. The managerial response to this shortage was rotational water distribution. Though meant to be equitable, in practice it is not, but serves to keep alive a clientele system under which the rich and the poor each remain in their current positions. The large farmers who grow sugarcane and rice are at the head of the system. They employ the wives and daughters of the tail-enders in their houses and farms and use this employment as leverage to influence the tail end farmers to grow the less remunerative 'dry' crops. In exchange the women keep their jobs and the poor farmers get enough water to grow their dry crops.

Source: Mollinga and van Straaten (1996).

The water scarcity that is resulting from lack of proper management of water resources has led to conflicts between Indian states and tensions between India and neighbouring countries, in particular Bangladesh and Pakistan. Conflicts between urban and rural users and between those who need water for different uses also increase and often lead to a worsened situation of the poorest and most marginal groups. In Maharashtra and Andhra Pradesh, for example, the use of groundwater for irrigated cash crops has brought many economic benefits to the families concerned. The womenfolk of landowners with irrigation pumps are able to use this water also for domestic purposes. Poor women found that their domestic shallow wells fell dry (Baldwin and Bhatnagar, 1996; Gandhigram Rural Institute, 1994; Rao, 1991) and they have become dependent on better-off farmers to use more distant irrigation wells for domestic purposes. The importance of these issues does, therefore, not only affect agricultural production, but also to the supply of drinking water, the reduction of poverty and the relations between states and with neighbouring countries.

IMPLEMENTATION OF THE SECTOR REFORMS

In Part II, research is presented on experiences with the implementation of the sector reforms for drinking water and sanitation. Chapters 5 to 7 are case studies of various institutional approaches to implement the sector reforms. Chapters 5 and 6 present two approaches, an independent registered support society and a NGO-supported community project in Gujarat. In chapter 5, K.P. Reddy first considers the effects of the water reform policy and its operationalization in Gujarat. He gives an interesting overview of the problems in the water sector in India and then presents a description of a model (WASMO), which could help to meet the challenges of rural water supply and sanitation in India. It can be compared with a model (in the sense of a suggested approach to the issues) presented in chapter 10 by A.J. James and P. Moriarty and the question will be raised under which conditions such models can work?

In Chapter 6, N. Barot gives convincing examples of community-built and -managed local water supply in Gujarat. The communities concerned received technical and financial assistance from NGOs without support from the government. She notes that effective services are rendered through a gender-balanced approach in planning and management. However, NGOs cannot do it alone. They do not have all the required capacities and funding. Although uniting forces may help, by itself the NGO sector cannot do enough to achieve sustained access for all. The question asked during the seminar was whether we can reconstruct the Indian water sector through NGOs? Is it not better feasible to involve local governments in a more systematic way?

Chapter 7 is a case study of community projects for village water supply or sanitation in Madhya Pradesh. They were supported by NGOs as part of the new government policy. Y. Kumar focusses in this chapter on the role of decentralization for the sanitation and drinking water sector. It turns out that important government services like the PHED do not have much trust in the capabilities of the community when it comes to water management! Under the

Government of India's (GoI) water sector reform financing, NGOs can act as moderators. However, in the case of village project planning, the district authorities finally decide. Kumar's evaluation of the experience in Madhya Pradesh is quite critical. Under GoI sector reform financing with PHED as moderator, there are no deadlines to meet, there is no accountability for the performance, and there are technical and procedural delays. Kumar finds no real devolution of funds and decisions to communities.

From ongoing research it has been learned that the technology and service levels used are very much linked to the scale of operations (Mollinga, 2003), the management structure and the available and known technologies (Blokland et al., 2002). Van Wijk (1997) distinguishes a number of alternative systems of community-based water supply in India, which can be taken as the point of departure and at the same time show the complicated nature of the problem: (1) communal water point services which provide water to whole habitations, often still without direct user management and payments; (2) group facilities, in which the users share the management and financing of the recurrent costs of a communal tap or hand pump; (3) community-managed vending kiosks, organized and operated by local groups or a private entrepreneur; (4) an autonomous local water distribution net managed by a community organization such as a water users' organization or a local water committee operating under the Panchayat, and (5) a small autonomous water supply operated, maintained and managed by the Panchayat, a water management committee, or a small Panchayat or private enterprise.

It seems useful to seek alternative approaches to satisfy the millennium water supply goals and the sanitation targets formulated in Johannesburg in August 2002 (for example Lettinga, 2002). Smet and van Wijk (2002) link the issue of technology of water supply with the specific needs of small communities in developing countries.

A number of issues remain important. Van Wijk et al. (2002) mention, for example:

(1) Newly constructed systems are not well maintained and non-use is high. Or, as Naidu (2002) formulates it: 'systems are falling into disrepair due to poor maintenance';
(2) Lack of integrated water management means that yields and water quality are declining. Naidu (2000) formulates it as water

shortages in summer months, sources drying up mainly due to depletion of groundwater; increasing incidence of water quality problems; damages due to recurring floods and droughts or other natural calamities; and increasing aspirations;

(3) Progress in rural sanitation has been much lower;
(4) User households have no say in these projects and women and poor people least of all.

Naidu (2002) concludes that unregulated and overexploited groundwater extraction has resulted in groundwater depletion and the resultant decline in water quality. When not managed better, this development threatens the sustainability of greater service access through decentralized water supplies, especially when many communities draw water for different uses from the same sources in an uncoordinated manner.

SCALING UP SECTOR REFORM

Part III of the book is devoted to scaling up the implementation of decentralized management of small water supplies by local government, user organizations and local enterprises in the light of the above-mentioned issues. In Chapter 8, pilot experiences and two large pilot projects are analysed. The first is Swajal in Uttar Pradesh, where a World Bank financed project unit supported community-managed water supply and sanitation projects on a competition basis, with Bank-contracted NGOs, CBOs and local consultancy groups as facilitators.

The second pilot project is the state sanitation programme in Kerala, in which case the state provides funds to all local councils based on an annual round of 'people's planning'. The availability of institutions that can meet the needs for training and other support services of the local councils and CBOs is one of the greatest bottlenecks in scaling up. C. Sijbesma concludes that the problem is not the principles of decentralization or water reform, but institutional support and adjustment is missing and there tends to be a continued focus on water supply. Among sector reformers the approach is still supplying new resources and not the better management of existing water resources. Under a pilot project for water sector reform, communities submit plans for new water supplies rather than for better management of available water. This emphasis will acerbate problems at watershed level as different sectors compete for same resources.

Chapter 9 describes and analyses the approach used to quickly identify demand and supply and bring the two together through a process of district scoping. The approach also serves to build up better knowledge and common understanding of the sector reforms. Chapter 10 presents a large number of cases of partnerships between local government (community councils and municipalities) and either private water societies or small entrepreneurs, showing how implementation is taking place in many states in India, from Andhra Pradesh, Karnataka, Kerala, and Maharashtra to Tamil Nadu and Uttaranchal.

COMPARISON WITH INTERNATIONAL TRENDS: PRIVATIZATION AND DELEGATION

In Part IV, the circle is closed by going back to the international context with attention to privatization of urban water supply and sanitation by national and multinational companies and to supranational policies on water resources management. Chapter 11 presents the Indian experiences with privatization of urban water supply and sanitation in India to national and international companies. The chapter presents the nature, status, and outcomes of 29 such cases in the period 1994-2003. V. Satyanarayana of the FIRE project in India presents possible improvements of urban water and wastewater services through private sector participation. The question was raised as to what the FIRE project can mean for the rural and peri-urban areas? Currently the project, which focusses on mobilizing private sector finance for infrastructure, has mainly experiences in the big cities in India.

Chapter 12 presents the water policies in Europe, their implementation in Germany and the Netherlands. M.P. van Dijk stresses the parallels and differences between India and the Netherlands. What are the lessons we can learn from each other? However, what works in Europe does not necessarily work in India. Examples are drawn from organizations in the water sector (water boards), environmental regulation (the role of EU norms) and financing the water sector (to a large extent with private sources in Europe). Chapter 13 summarizes the findings, draws conclusions, and suggests an agenda for further research.

It is concluded that the lack of success of sector reform is grounded in problems of political and institutional change. The attitudes of government bureaucracy and (para) statal utilities leave much to be desired. Both are unwilling to let go their 100 per cent control over the sector, while they are unable to implement the necessary reforms themselves. Sub-issues are that villagers need information and technical assistance, but at present the utilities in the sector do not want to work with NGOs. However, they do not have themselves the capacity and numbers of staff necessary for the kind of support needed.

Fortunately, powerful political and institutional lobbies cause changes in policies in certain states. Barot for Gujarat and Sijbesma for Kerala give examples of progress. Often the state and central governments think differently about the place of community-managed, small-size systems in the overall water policy. An example is the Narmada project and the Indian river-linking programme. The latter is at the moment a mega-scheme mainly pushed by the centre. Consequently, water demand management within the water sector as a whole is not addressed in policies and implementation programmes. The conclusion is drawn that there exists no real integrated water resource management in India because of multiple institutions and lack of coordination. A lot can be improved and this book may help to work in the right direction.

RESEARCH IDEAS

The relevance of research in the domestic water supply sector in India is high. India has the second largest population in the world and is the world's largest democracy. The sector reforms linked to the country-wide (re)establishment of local government is the greatest change in India since the adoption of the free supply of safe water for rural areas in 1972. Many other countries undertake similar decentralization and devolution of water and sanitation to local levels, but in India the scale is many times larger. The most important research question is: What happens during the operationialization of water policies in India? What is of global relevance from this experience? The degree of success or failure will impact conditions in India as well as globally.

A very convincing example is furthermore set when a large and complex country such as India successfully decentralizes its water supply and sanitation to institutions at the local level in such ways that safe water and sanitation reach all its citizens and continue to serve them well. In this light, it is surprising that the country does not yet have an organized research programme on the processes and effects of the sector reforms.

This book shows that important lessons can be learned to help improve implementation, especially in the fields of effective support organizations for locally managed water supply and sanitation. Other areas for research are ways to establish effective partnerships with small and local private enterprises, analysis of impacts from large privatizations for service delivery and costs for the poor, effects of measures for more effective management of water demands and research on linkages between community-managed water supply and sanitation and the integrated management of the water resources on which the communities depend. It is hoped that this book, with its richness of information on experiences with different actors, will stimulate the emergence of such a research agenda. There are also some issues that have not been dealt with, in particular, water and sanitation in the urban areas.

WATER ISSUES IN THE URBAN AREAS

Water issues in the urban areas are also important as described for example in Zerah (2000) for Delhi. Specific urban problems are floods of the rivers, which cause problems for the slums built on the river banks (for an example in Ahmedabad, see Pangotra and Shukla, 1994) and the increasing pollution of water sources which require water to be brought in from increasingly large distances. Bangalore is a typical case of an Indian city struggling with water supply. At a small scale it has started to clean up its tanks (Ulsoor tank clean-up, see *Deccan Herald*, 8 December 2002), but at a larger scale the city has realized that groundwater legislation needs to be changed to increase the potential of the available water in India in general and Bangalore in particular.[1] Although the Central Ground Water Authority, set up as per Supreme Court's directive, has improved the situation, there remains an important problem. This concerns the enforceability of the authority's directives, which depends largely on the responsiveness of the states. In the current situation, parts of the city are not connected to the drinking water grid. Although not allowed without permission, the inhabitants are forced to dig bore holes, which mean a lowering of the water table.[2] Alternatively the poor depend on water vendors and water trucks of the municipality. The result is that water quality in Bangalore is beginning to become doubtful (see Box 1.6).

Box 1.6: Drinking Water Supply Problems in Bangalore

According to the *Times of India* (10 December 2002): 'the administration has been unable to make provisions for clean drinking water in many new suburbs. . . . The Ground Water Board in 1998 marked many areas in north Bangalore and Whitefield as "dark blocks", where there had been more than 85 per cent over-utilization. In some areas it was as much as 141 per cent. In many places water from damaged underground sewage pipes leaked into ground water contaminating it with poisonous substances'.

However, even the surface water is not safe. There were over one hundred lakes in the city, but most have disappeared over the years due to commercial building activities. The ones that have remained have water that's highly contaminated, because many drains in the area pump waste water into the lakes. Poor solid waste management adds to all this.

The Tata Environmental Resources Institute (TERI) has done pilot projects with two residents' associations in Bangalore involving school children, but the city could do with much more than pilot studies. TERI's recommendations are summarized in Box 1.7.

The State Government of Karnataka is contemplating handing over urban drinking water supply to private operators. The chief minister is very much interested in addressing the existing system, which has many lapses in this way (*Times of India*, 20 December 2002). The Ahmedabad water supply has been studied by Suhane (1998). He finds that by 1991 only 85 per cent of the urban population had access to safe drinking water. The average availability in the slums is only half of what is available in the Class 4 towns in Gujarat

Box 1.7: Suggestions of TERI to Improve the Situation in Bangalore

Rainwater harvesting programmes to recharge the lakes and tanks;
Groundwater recharging programmes through the use of special points and cleaning of sewer waste;
Reclamation of lakes and tanks;
In areas where there are underground drainage systems segregation of sewage is essential;
Development of separate landfills in the city;
A separate landfill for medical waste;
Connection of underground water systems to sewage pipes;
Segregation of organic and inorganic waste;
Recycling of plastic and paper;
Setting up incinerators and compost sites; and
Banning of plastic carry bags for food items.

and slightly more than 50 per cent of the desirable limit of 40 l per consumer per day. Other shocking statistics are the number of persons per water connection (14.5) and the daily hours of water supply (3.5 per day) in Ahmedabad. He notes as major problems:

(1) The concept of cost recovery, which is not taken seriously by the different agencies;
(2) A low proportion of meter connections; and
(3) Supply constraints which have limited the expansion of the networks and sanctioning of new connections.

Although of great importance to economic and social development in India, the authors of this book have however chosen to concentrate on research related to drinking water supply and sanitation of the rural and peri-urban populations. The reason is that, as documented in several of the chapters, these groups still constitute the largest proportion of the Indian people and that for them, access to reliable water supply and improved sanitation is still worse than for the urban majority.

CONCLUSIONS

All, poor, rural and urban, have the right to sustainable and equitable water and sanitation services. This is an enormous challenge for most developing countries and certainly the densely populated countries of South Asia. The objectives of the proposed workshop were:

- To bring together a group of Indian and Dutch researchers on rural and peri-urban water supply and sanitation with special expertise in poverty and social equity aspects;
- To review the priority issues that promote/hamper the access of the rural and peri-urban poor to sustainable and equitable water supply and sanitation provision;
- To identify areas and topics of research that can contribute to equitable and sustained access of the poor to good water and sanitation (set a tentative agenda);
- To assess where Indian key sector officials and other researchers would like to cooperate; and
- To plan follow-up activities to establish research partnerships and design and plan research activities based on mutual interest in and commitment to the challenge at stake.

The workshop shed light on factors explaining the success and failures of different approaches of dealing with water for the poor. In particular, the experiences of different departments and donors with programmes dealing with poor people have been analysed. The main questions that emerged from the workshop regarding research on the water and sanitation sector in India were:

(1) What is the importance and potential of different management structures in the water and sanitation sector, raised by Blokland et al. (2000, 2002), amongst others and reported on in this book by Reddy, Barot and Kumar;
(2) Which technologies have been tried in the rural and peri-urban areas? Besides the work of Chakravarty (1990) and Jal Manthan (2002), an impression can be gained from the works of Reddy and Dev (this book) and van Wijk (2002 and this book);
(3) What are the specific problems in the peri-urban areas? Reference can here be made to James et al. (2002) and James and Moriarty (this book) and Suhane (1998);
(4) What is the experience with PPPs in financing and developing the water and sanitation sector? Examples that are referred to

are FIRE (1998) and van Dijk (2002) and an analysis of 29 cases by Satyaranaranya in this book; and

(5) What are the different sources of finance for research, projects and programmes in this sector? In this book, Satyaranaranya addresses mobilizing private capital for public services. One option is using the Municipal bond market for urban infrastructure. Ahmedabad is one of the first cities that actually did this in India (FIRE, 1999) and further study is needed to see if such solutions equally benefit the poor.

The overriding aim of the water sector in India is to reach the millennium goals for water supply and the Johannesburg goals concerning the sanitation sector. This requires a concerted effort, including a contribution from joint research to better understand the issues. There are lots of issues in the water sector in India. Some are of a political nature, such as the quarrels between states such as Tamil Nadu, Andhra Pradesh and Karnataka. Indians call this hydropolitics and refer to the two states locked in a complex range of disputes over irrigation projects across the Krishna River (*Indian Express*, 29 June 2001 and Mollinga, 2003). Another conflict concerns the project supplying water to Chennai, the capital of Tamil Nadu, known as the multi-crore Veeranam water project, which is also troubled by accusations of bad governance (*Hindu*, 7 December 2002). Summing up, the main issues are:

- *Political problems*: Between different states, which are the responsibility of the Central Water Commission, but come with a lot of political rhetoric and may lead to case at the High Court as in the case of Karnataka;
- *Governance issues*: Different ministries are involved at the Central level: the Water Resources Ministry, Ministry for Rural Development, Ministry of Urban Affairs and Employment (for O&M of urban water supply and sanitation systems). The issue of transparency also came up in some of the examples given in the text. Integrated water resources management demands a new framework within which there may be a need for changes in the existing interactions between politics, laws, regulations, institutions and civil society;
- *Management issues*: A lot of infrastructure has been put in place

but is not properly used and maintained. Water utilities resist the changes and are reluctant to develop the expertise and attitudes required for water and sanitation under the new legislation;

- *Social issues*: How to reach the poor and how to involve the people concerned with gender and social equality? In this respect, Sunshine (2002) speaks of the 'denial of community control of water resources';
- *Technological issues*: What are the best technologies to achieve the drinking water supply and sanitation goals under decentralized public management, private management and combinations of the two;
- *Financial issues*: Which systems can be introduced which are self-financing *and* equitable for the poor;
- *Environmental issues*: In particular, pollution of freshwater resources and how to reach ecosystem sustainability in the context of multi-purpose and often conflicting uses of water increasing water demands and decentralization of water management?
- *Water management issues*: Inadequate efforts to conserve water, to use it efficiently and to allow recharge of the groundwater;
- *Institutional issues*: Which organizations can support the local governments and user groups of rural and urban poor to maintain, manage, upgrade and, where needed, newly install the service mix that they want and can afford.

Those participating in the seminar identified areas and topics on which they would like to cooperate in future. The remaining topics, 'to assess where Indian key sector officials and other researchers would like to cooperate' and 'to plan follow-up activities to establish research partnerships and design and plan research activities based on mutual interest in and commitment to the challenge at stake' were pursued further at a follow-up meeting in Hyderabad, India, in July 2003.

NOTES

1. The water rights under Common Law in India consider groundwater not as a common resource but as belonging to the landowner.
2. Uncontrolled use of bore well technology has allowed groundwater to be extracted at rates exceeding groundwater recharge.

REFERENCES

Baldwin, Jim A. and Sudhir N. Bhatnagar, 'Sustainability through Training', in John Pickford et al. (eds.) *Reaching the Unreached, Challenges for the 21st Century: Proceedings of the 22nd WEDC Conference, New Delhi, India, 9–13 September 1996*, Loughborough, UK: Water, Engineering and Development Centre, Loughborough University of Technology, 1996, pp. 24–6.

Blokland, M., O. Braadbaart and K. Schwartz, *The Public Water PLC*, Delft: IHE, 2000.

Blokland, M., L. Saade and M.P. van Dijk, 'Insitutional Arrangements for Municipal Wastewater and Sanitation', Geneva: WSSCC-IMO, 2002.

Chakravaty, S., *Drinking Water and Science, An Indian Experiment*, New Delhi: Batra Book Service, 1990.

Dahn Foundation, A Conference on Tanks, Madurai: Dahn Foundation, 2002.

Dijk, M.P. van, 'The Role of Financial Institutions and Markets in Urban Development in India, with Examples from Karnataka and Gujarat' Lecture for high-level delegation of Indian government, Rotterdam: IHS, 2002.

Dijk, M.P. van and N.G. Schulte Nordholt (eds.), 'Privatisation Experiences in Africa and Asia', Amsterdam: SISWO, 1994.

FIRE, 'Pune Water Supply and Sewerage Project: Focus on PSP', New Delhi: FIRE Project, 1998.

———, 'The Municipal Bond Market for Urban Infrastructure', New Delhi: FIRE Project, 1999, pp. 1–23.

Gandhigram Rural Institute, 'Sand over the Soil: PRA Approach for Sorting Out an Incessant Agricultural Problem in a Western Ghat Village', in *RRA Notes,* no. 19, London: International Institute for Environment and Development, Sustainable Agriculture Programme, 1994.

Jal Manthan, 'A Rural Think Tank', New Delhi: Watsan Programme South Asia, 2002.

James, A.J., J. Verhagen, C. van Wijk, R. Nanavaty, M. Parikh and M. Bhatt, 'Transforming Time into Money Using Water: A Participatory Study of Economics and Gender in Rural India', Delft: IRC, 2002.

Kolsky, P., E. Baumann, J. Chilton, R. Bhatia and C. van Wijk, 'Evaluation of Unicef Water and Environmental Sanitation Activities in India, 1966–1998', New Delhi: UNICEF, 1999.

Lettinga, G., 'Rioleringskunde op z'n westers', in *Volkskrant*, 28 October 2002.

Loon, F.D. van and M.P. van Dijk, 'The Financial Flows to and Capital Markets in Asia', in K. Fukasaku (ed.), *Regional Co-operation and Integration in Asia*, Paris: OECD, 1995, pp. 175–93.

Mehta, Supriya Prabhu, 'Planning Solutions to Reduce Flood Vulnerability of Low-income Settelements: A Case Study of Riverbed Settlements in Ahmedabad, India', Research thesis, Bangkok: AIT, 1999.

Mollinga, P.P., *On the Water Front, Water Distribution Technology and Agrarian Change in a South Indian Canal Irrigation System*, Hyderabad: Orient Longman, 2003.

Mollinga, P.P. and C.J.M. van Straaten, 'The Politics of Water Distribution: Negotiating Resource Use in a South Indian Canal Irrigation System', in Peter Howsam, and Richard Carter (eds.), *Water Policy: Allocation and Management in Practice*, London, E. and F.N. Spon, 1996, pp. 244–50.

Naidu, V., *Indian Reforms Initiatives in the Water Sector*, Washington: World Bank Water Forum, 2002.

Pangotra, P. and P.R. Shukla, *Management Plan for River Sabarmati*, Ahmedabad: School of Planning, 1994.

Put, M. and M.P. van Dijk, 'Semi-arid Indian Agriculture, Land, Water and Crop Management in Southern India', in *Bulletin 316*, Amsterdam: Royal Tropical Institute, 1989.

Put, M. and M.P. van Dijk (eds.), *Government and NGOs Interventions in Dry Land Agriculture, A Study of Two Projects in Andhra Pradesh*, New Delhi: Manohar, 2000.

Rao, Brinda, 'Women and Water in Rural Maharashtra', in *Environment and Urbanization*, vol. 3, no. 2, 1991, pp. 57-65.

Suhane, R., 'Dynamics of Water Supply Management System, A Case of Ahmedabad', Master's thesis, Ahmedabad: School of Planning, 1998.

Sinha, S., 'Return to Equity, Financial Structure and Risk Contracting in Infrastructure Projects', in *Vikalpa*, vol. 20, no. 4, 1995, pp. 11–21.

Smet, J. and C. van Wijk, 'Small Community Water Supplies: Technology, People and Partnerships', Technical paper no. 40, Delft: IRC, 2002.

Sunshine Spartel, T., 'Influence of Soci-cultural Norms on the Sustainability of Rural Water Supply and Sanitation, A Case Study of Tamil Nadu', M.Sc. thesis, Guelp: University, 2002.

Wijk, C. van, 'Constraints and Key Approaches in Water Supply and Sanitation for Low Income Urban Neighbourhoods', New Delhi: Task Force on O&M of Urban Water Supply and Sanitation Systems, 1997.

Wijk, Christine van, Prathap K. Reddy and Thresiamma Mathew, 'Water Supply, Sanitation and Rural Poverty Reduction in Gujarat and Kerala States', The Hague: Institute of Social Studies, 2002.

WASH, 'WASH for Gujarat Relief and Rehabilitation', Geneva: WSSCC, 2002.

World Bank, 'A Water Resources Management Sector Review Report for Urban Water Supply and Sanitation, Washington, June 1998.

———, 'A Water Resources Management Sector Review Report for Rural Water Supply and Sanitation in India, Washington, January 1998.

———, 'Water and Work for India's Poorest Rural Region', Washington: IBRD project brief, 1998c.

WSSCC, 'WASH in Gujarat', Geneva: WSSCC, 2002.

Zerah, M.H., *Water: Unreliable Supply in Delhi*, New Delhi: Manohar, 2002.

CHAPTER 2

Groundwater Resources in India: The National Water Policy

J.S. BURJIA

INTRODUCTION

As water is vital for existence of life, the government is expected to play an important role in ensuring its availability and sustainability. Under the Constitution of India, the subject 'Water' has been placed in the State List. The Ministry of Water Resources, Government of India, is, however, responsible for laying down the policy guidelines for the country's water resources. The following are the main functions assigned to the Ministry of Water Resources (GoI, 2003):

(1) Overall planning, policy formulation, coordination and guidance in the sector of water resources;
(2) Coordination, mediation and facilitation in regard to the resolution of differences or disputes relating to inter-state rivers and overseeing of the implementation of inter-state projects;
(3) Overall planning for the development of groundwater resources, assessment of utilizable resources and formulation of policies of exploitation, overseeing of and support to the state-level activities in groundwater development;
(4) Regulation of groundwater extraction and creation of general awareness of the need and steps for artificial recharge in view of the depletion of the resource;
(5) Formulation of the national water development perspective and determination of the water balance of different basins/ sub-basins for possible inter-basin transfers;
(6) Overall policy formulation, planning and guidance in respect of minor irrigation and command area development, and also the administration and monitoring of the centrally sponsored schemes in these areas;

(7) Operation of the central network for flood forecasting and warning on important rivers, the provision of central assistance for some state schemes in special cases and preparation of flood control master plans for the Ganga and the Brahmaputra River systems;
(8) Infrastructural, technical and research support for sectoral development at the state-level.

For achieving the desired goals, the national water policy was revised in 2002 (GoI, 2002). It has now been adopted by the National Water Resources Council, which is headed by the prime minister of India and consists of the chief ministers of all the states and the lt. governors of union territories (GoI, 2003). The national water policy recognizes water as a precious national asset. It embodies the nation's resolve that planning, development and management of water resources would be governed by the nation's overall development perspectives.

HIGHLIGHTS OF THE NEW POLICY

The National Water Policy, 2002, emphasizes the integrated development and management of India's water resources for the optimal and sustainable utilization of the available surface and groundwater, the creation of a well-developed information system, the use of traditional methods of water conservation, and the development and use of non-conventional methods for water utilization and demand management. The revised policy integrates quantity and quality aspects as well as environmental considerations for water through adequate institutional arrangements. Furthermore, 'ecological needs' have been assigned due priority in the allocation of water to the various sectors. Greater emphasis has been laid on water quality aspects. The policy also stresses involvement of people in project planning and a participatory approach in water resources management. The salient features of the National Water Policy, 2002, are the following (GoI, 2002):

- Water is a precious natural resource and its planning, development and management should be governed by national perspectives;

- A well-developed information system for water-related data at national/state level should be established with a network of databanks and databases integrating and strengthening the existing central and state-level agencies;
- The basis for planning water resources development and management is the hydrological unit such as a river basin or sub-basin. Appropriate river basin organizations should be established for the planned development and management of the river basins;
- Water should be made available to water-short areas by transfer from other areas, including transfer from one river basin to another, after taking into account the requirements of the areas/ basins;
- Planning of water resources development projects should, as far as possible, be for multi-purpose projects with an integrated and multi-disciplinary approach having regard to human and ecological aspects, including those of disadvantaged sections of the society;
- Drinking water has been assigned the first priority in the allocation of water;
- The exploration of groundwater should be regulated with reference to recharge possibilities and considerations of social equity. The detrimental environmental consequences of over-exploitation of groundwater need to be effectively prevented;
- Careful planning is necessary to ensure that construction and rehabilitation activities proceed simultaneously. A skeletal national policy on resettlement and rehabilitation needs to be formulated so that project-affected persons share the benefits through proper rehabilitation;
- Adequate emphasis needs to be given to the physical and financial sustainability of existing water resources facilities. There is a need to ensure that the water charges for various uses are fixed in such a way as to cover initially at least the operation and maintenance costs and subsequently a part of the capital costs;
- The management of the water resources for the different uses should incorporate a participatory approach by involving users and other stakeholders, along with various governmental agencies, in an effective and decisive manner;

- Both surface water and groundwater should be regularly monitored for quality. Effluents should be treated to acceptable levels and standards before discharging them into natural streams. Minimum flows should be ensured in the perennial streams for maintaining their ecological balance;
- The efficiency in the utilization of water should be improved with regard to all possible uses and conservation consciousness promoted through education, regulation, incentives and disincentives;
- There should be a master plan for flood control and a management system for each flood-prone basin. In flood control and management, the strategy should be to reduce the intensity of floods;
- Land erosion by the sea or rivers should be minimized through suitable cost-effective measures. Indiscriminate occupation of, and economic activities in, coastal areas and flood plain zones should be regulated;
- The needs of drought-prone areas should be given priority in the planning of projects for the development of water resources. These areas should be made less vulnerable through various measures;
- Water sharing/distribution amongst the states should be guided by a national perspective with due regard to water resources availability and needs within the concerned river basins;
- Training and research efforts should be intensified as an integral part of water resources development.

The action plan for the implementation of the national water policy had been adopted in a meeting of central ministries and state governments in February 2003. The National Water Policy, 2002 has set the water allocation priorities as follows:

(1) Drinking water
(2) Irrigation
(3) Hydropower
(4) Ecology
(5) Agro-industries and non-agricultural industries
(6) Navigation and other uses.

Not only has drinking water been given first priority in the national water policy, but the policy also states that irrigation and multipurpose projects should invariably include a drinking water component wherever there is no alternative source of drinking water.

GROUNDWATER DEPLETION

According to the available data, there is a heavy dependence on groundwater for irrigation and particularly for drinking water in rural and semi-urban areas. Groundwater meets 85 per cent of the drinking water needs of rural India and sustains 60 per cent of the irrigated agriculture. Over the last five decades, the volume of groundwater-based irrigation has increased nine times. In 1951, an area of 6.5 mha was irrigated from groundwater sources and this has now increased to more than 50.0 mha. More than 17 million wells all over the country are providing irrigation water to more than 60 per cent of the irrigated area. Table 2.1 depicts the increasing stress on groundwater in the last 50 years.

The rapid increase in the development of groundwater resources has undoubtedly contributed to the expansion of irrigated agriculture and the overall economic development in the country and has improved the quality of life in India. In the above-given period of time, food production has increased, the pace of industrial development has accelerated, and the drinking water needs of a growing population and water needs for a rapidly increased urbanization have been met to a large extent. The use of the national groundwater resources has contributed substantially to all these developments.

Table 2.1: Numbers of Water Supply Systems Relying on Groundwater between 1951 and 1992

	1951	1992
Dug wells	3.86 million	10.12 million
Shallow tube wells	3,000	5.38 million
Public bore/tube wells	Negligible	68,000
Electric pump sets	Negligible	9.34 million
Diesel pump sets	66,000	4.59 million

On the one hand, we need to keep up the pace of development, and agricultural production needs to be increased to feed the growing population. It has been observed that the increasing dependency on groundwater for irrigation is depleting the groundwater resources. Depletion of groundwater has already adversely affected the availability and supply of drinking water. The groundwater levels have gone down in many parts of the country. According to the most recent survey conducted by the Central Ground Water Board (CGWB), 310 blocks in the country are withdrawing more groundwater than is naturally replenished and about 160 blocks are withdrawing groundwater at a rate of between 85–100 per cent of its natural replenishment. The situation is alarming and needs to be addressed with the utmost priority.

Given this critical situation, action is required on many fronts to manage the situation. Broadly, the required steps can be listed under three major categories: conservation, regulation and augmentation.

Conservation

The following steps are considered necessary in this regard:

(1) With groundwater for irrigation in the country now taking up over 60 per cent of the total water use for agriculture, there is an urgent need for a change of irrigation practices so that groundwater resources can be kept intact for drinking water requirements;
(2) Alternative irrigation technologies such as drip and sprinkler irrigation need to be developed and popularized;
(3) Agricultural practices need to be changed. For example, agricultural scientists need to develop varieties which require less water;
(4) Another important action area is raising public awareness of the scarcity of this economic resource. At present, the Groundwater Board has 150 mass awareness programmes (GoI, 2003). These programmes require the involvement of social scientists and researchers not only in development, but also in independent evaluation, if possible together with consumer organizations and other representatives of stakeholders such as farmers and women;

(5) It has been observed that the rate of leakage in the conveyor systems is high, especially in the case of dug canals. The canals should, therefore, be lined;
(6) People sometimes leave the water taps open. Researchers need to work on this to find out the extent of loss and suggest remedial measures;
(7) At present, waste water is not treated and recycled for reuse. When local governments and municipalities take up this issue as a priority, freshwater, which is now used for irrigating gardens and so on could be saved for drinking water purposes.

Regulatory Measures

Another important area for conservation is regulatory intervention. The Central Ground Water Authority (CGWA), constituted in 1997 under the directions of the Supreme Court of India, is entrusted with the regulation and control of groundwater development and its management throughout the country. The CGWA has notified 11 areas in the country where construction of new structures for the withdrawal of groundwater have been banned. Although these areas have been notified, questions are being raised about the enforceability of the directions. The Authority does not have its own machinery to enforce application. For this purpose, it depends on the state government machinery.

Keeping in view the critical situation in various parts of the country, there is a need not only to strengthen the regulatory mechanisms, but also to take various other steps to bring about some discipline in the exploitation of groundwater resources. Therefore, researchers need to work in this area to find out what the effects are of the ban imposed in the notified areas and to suggest additional measures, which may be taken to deal with the situation.

Augmentation of Groundwater Resources

In India, most of the rain falls during some three months of the year, with the result that the monsoon run-off that is wasted is quite substantial. The total precipitation in the country is around 4,000 billion cubic metres (BCM). The amount that is currently available in the form of surface water or replenished groundwater is put at

1,869 BCM. There is much scope for the further utilization of surplus run-off for surface and groundwater storage. Therefore, artificial recharge and rainwater harvesting are considered very important to augment the water resources, particularly in those areas where the exploitation of groundwater surpasses its natural replenishment.

The CGWB and CGWA popularize rainwater harvesting with simple techniques which utilize surplus monsoon run-off for artificial recharge of groundwater in the country. Since a large number of schemes needs to be taken up throughout the country, this needs public cooperation and participation, and for this, people need to be educated, trained and made more aware. The utilization of surplus run-off is also considered necessary to arrest sea water ingression in coastal areas.

In fact, for the augmentation of groundwater and for taking up rainwater harvesting schemes throughout the country, awareness and people's participation are necessary at every level. It should become a mass movement if the groundwater resources are to be made sustainable. Local government organizations and municipalities also need to be involved in taking up schemes and in the evaluation and impact assessment of artificial recharge interventions. A critical issue in this respect is the balancing of control, duties and rights between the government and the user communities (Mahesh and Subramaniam, 2004).

One of the important areas in water augmentation is rooftop rainwater harvesting. Local government organizations and municipalities could make rooftop rainwater harvesting mandatory for future constructions and give some incentives to existing building owners in the shape of a rebate in house tax to enable/encourage them to construct rooftop rainwater harvesting structures.

The need for addressing drinking water requirements is of paramount importance. Where the groundwater levels are being depleted, the position becomes very critical. It becomes, therefore, even more necessary to make augmentation measures a priority in critical geographic areas.

The CGWB is a scientific organization under the Ministry of Water Resources. It generates data through the exploration of groundwater resources and is involved in testing the quality of groundwater. Based on these data, the Board prepares district maps and other documents on groundwater resources. The CGWB has started the process of digitalizing the groundwater maps for all the districts of the country. Fifteen such maps have already been released. These digitalized maps will be put on the organization's website for the information of the public.

These maps provide valuable information which can help in the planning and development of groundwater resources in each area. The maps can be used as basic decision-making tools for forward planning. The maps can also be used for taking up artificial recharge schemes in areas where groundwater aquifers are depleting at a fast rate and the saline ingress is likely to take place in the coastal areas. Social researchers can work further on this and suggest ways by which the information on the groundwater situation generated by the CGWB can be put to gainful use by the public and to avoid exploitation by powerful groups.

WATER QUALITY ASPECTS

Quality aspects are equally important in the issues relating to drinking water. The National Water Policy, 2002 stresses that both surface and groundwater should be regularly monitored for quality and a phased programme should be undertaken for the improvement of the water quality. In the Ministry of Water Resources, the Central Water Commission regularly monitors the country's major rivers for hydrological data and water quality. The CGWB monitors groundwater levels and quality year-round with the help of a network of 15,000 monitoring stations in the country.

Broadly speaking, groundwater contamination takes place from two sources: natural, e.g. arsenic, iron, and fluoride, and manmade, e.g. through industrial activities and overexploitation of groundwater leading to intrusion of saline water or water of a poor quality. In canal command areas, for example, salinity increase due to water logging is common, while in coastal regions, salinity ingress takes place because of overextraction of groundwater. In order to ensure safe drinking water, we should develop cost effective and environmentally friendly water treatment plants for the removal of arsenic and fluoride. Safe designs for urban waste disposal, including landfill designs, and the development of technologies for recycling and reuse of solid waste should be developed. Inland desalinization plants with provisions for the safe disposal of effluents also need to be taken up in the affected areas.

Communities have to be made conscious about water quality through health education and awareness campaigns and water testing kits have to be made available to a range of institutions, including schools and colleges and qualified NGOs in the area. All possible measures should be taken to remove the disparity in access to potable water across regions and socio-economic groups. A system of guarantee periods and random checks should be developed to detect poor quality construction. The choice of technology in case of schemes related to water quality, including for the detection of fluoride, iron, and arsenic, should become district/block specific. Further research is required to improve the available technologies for treatment of chemically contaminated water, in terms of their simplification and increased cost effectiveness.

CONCLUSION

It can be said that the serious situation regarding the availability and quality of water in India calls for a greater research contribution. Research is needed to more effectively reduce water losses in agriculture and develop and adopt crop varieties that require less water. Affordable and effective methods have to be developed and tested that raise the awareness on water scarcity and lead to countervailing practices and measures. Research is also needed to measure the effects of the ban on groundwater withdrawal, test other measures for regulation, and investigate ways of spreading the use of rainwater harvesting. Social research can help the CGWB develop and test strategies to stimulate wider access to and beneficial use of the groundwater data, to protect drinking water and counteract exploitation for purposes that threaten the priorities laid down in the Indian national policy and legal rulings.

REFERENCES

Government of India, National Water Policy, New Delhi: Ministry of Water Resources, http://wrmin.nic.in/policy/nwp2002.pdf, 2002.

———, Fourth Editors Conference on Social Sector Issues, New Delhi: Ministry of Water Resources, http://wrmin.nic.in/editors-conference.pdf, 28 August 2003.

Mahesh, Ashwin and Vincent Subramaniam, 'Bypassing Community Rights', in *India Together*, http://indiatogether.org/environment/water/nwp.htm, April 2004.

CHAPTER 3

Financial and Economic Sustainability: Public–Private Partnership

U. SANKAR

INTRODUCTION

Until recently, the public sector in India was assigned a dominant role in the planning, development and management of drinking water supply and sanitation projects. This paper explores the sustainability of this approach and its alternative of public–private partnerships (PPP). In section two, it gives reasons for assigning a dominant role for the government in the past, assesses the current status of drinking water supply, and sanitation in rural areas in terms of their availability, type of access and quality, and highlights the problems in continuing the centralized supply-driven approach. Section three argues a case for decentralized demand-driven approach based on PPP. It identifies the roles for government, private firms and local communities in planning, development and management of drinking water supply and sanitation projects. It considers problems of coordination, cost sharing, pricing, access to the poor and economic sustainability. Two examples of public–private partnership are given in section four to illustrate issues in the design and implementation of PPP. Section five contains concluding remarks.

DRINKING WATER SUPPLY AND SANITATION: PAST POLICY AND CURRENT STATUS

Dominant Role for Public Water Supply

The Government of India and the state governments have, in the past, assigned a dominant role for the public sector in the provision of drinking water and sanitation services. The reasons are partly based on the nature and characteristics of the good/service and partly on the belief that the public provision can correct market failures and achieve social goals.

Water is a natural resource. Water resources such as rivers, canals, ponds, lakes and streams are common property resources with open access. The public trust doctrine rests on the principle that common property resources which are important to the people as a whole should not be a subject of private ownership. The state is to act as the trustee of the natural resource. Groundwater in private lands is a common-pool resource. Most governments give owners of lands only the right to extract water for private use.

Drinking water and sanitation services are viewed as merit goods. Merit goods are those that are in the nature of private goods in that their consumption may not be non-rival but yet the amounts provided by the market may not be to the extent that the community would like. Some would argue that these communal wants transcend individual preferences. Water is also a basic need; it is an important means of life support. The Supreme Court of India, in its various decisions, has stressed the citizens' right to a wholesome environment which includes access to safe drinking water and clean air. As an essential good, the price elasticity of demand for drinking water is low. Hence, many governments favour provision of drinking water to poor at affordable prices.

Water supply and sanitation services are regarded as public utility services. In case of a water supply system, there may be significant economies of scale in storage of water and treatment of water. One can also avoid duplication of facilities by having a monopoly. A public monopoly also provides an opportunity for provision of services to poor, either at subsidized prices with government bearing the cost of subsidy, or cross-subsidization of poor by rich, while ensuring reasonable return on the investments. Subsidy/cross-subsidy is preferred to achieve goals such as equity (affordable prices to poor), provision of merit goods (meeting minimum needs), and realizing external benefits (savings in health costs because of safe drinking water and good sanitation services).

If the public utilities are managed efficiently in the sense of providing the services at least social costs, and achieving the goals of equity and balanced regional development, and economic sustainability, then there is a case for a dominant role for public sector in the provision of water supply and sanitation services. Let us see to what extent the expectations have been realized.

Current Status of Rural Water Supply and Sanitation

The two main sources of data on the present conditions of drinking water and sanitation at the national level are: (a) the National Sample Survey, 54th round conducted during January–June 1998, available in NSSO (1999), and (b) Census of India conducted in February 2001, available with the Registrar General of India (2003).

Earlier rounds of NSS, 28th round (October 1973–June 1974), 38th round (January–December 1983), 44th round (July 1988–June 1989), and 49th round (January–June 1993) contain data relating to conditions of drinking water or/and sanitation. The 54th round of the NSS survey is based on a larger sample; it also provides new information. The National Sample Survey Organization (NSSO) gives information about source, availability, right of use, distance from source, supplementary sources and quality of drinking water; type, right of use and distance from the place for bathroom and latrine; and a few indicators of hygiene (GoI, 1999). The 2001 Census gives information about sources and distances from households for drinking water, and availability and types of bathrooms and latrines (Registrar General of India, 2003).

Table 3.1 gives the percentage distribution of households by principal source of drinking water during January–June 1998. According to the NSSO (GoI, 1999), the source tap refers to 'the supply of water to the households through pipe after suitable treatment, if required, by corporation, municipality, Panchayat or other local authorities, or any private or public housing estate or water treating agency' (p. 6). Of the eight sources mentioned, only this source provides treated water. It may be noted that tap was the principal source for 18.7 per cent of rural households and 70.1 per cent of urban households. The shares of tubewell, hand pump and wells were 75.9 per cent in rural areas and 28.0 per cent in urban areas. Common property resources like tanks, ponds, rivers, canals, lakes and springs were principal source for 4.9 per cent of rural households and 0.6 per cent of urban households.

Table 3.1: Percentage Distributions of Households by Principal Source of Drinking Water during January–June 1998

Source of Drinking Water	Percentage of Households	
	Rural	Urban
Tap	18.7	70.1
Tube well/hand pump	50.1	21.3
Well	25.8	6.7
Tank/pond reserved for drinking	1.3	0.2
Other tank/pond	0.6	0.1
River/canal/lake	1.3	0.2
Spring	1.7	0.1
Tanker	0.2	1.0
Other	0.2	0.1
All	100.0	100.0

Source: GoI–NSSO (1999), Table 1, p. 22.

Apart from the rural-urban disparity at the national level, there are wide regional variations between poor states and rich states in the distributions of households by principal source of water supply in rural areas. Based on the work by the World Bank (2003), we have chosen four poor states with a per capita annual income of Rs. 7,500 or less during 1997–2000, and four rich states with a per capita annual income of Rs. 15,000 or more during 1997–2000, for a comparative assessment of the principal source of drinking water supply. The poor states were Bihar, Orissa, UP and Assam and the rich states were Maharashtra, Punjab, Haryana and Gujarat. In all four poor states, less than 9 per cent of the rural households had tap as a principal source. In Bihar, the state with the lowest per capita annual income of Rs. 24,500 less than 1 per cent of the rural households had tap as a principal source. In the four rich states, the percentage of rural households with tap as a principal source ranged from 14.8 in Punjab to 46.6 in Gujarat (Table 3.2).

Both the NSS and the census provide information about the type of access measured in terms of distance from the principal source. NSS results for rural and urban areas are given in Table 3.3.

In rural areas, less than one-ninth of households had access to principal water source within dwelling, but the corresponding figure for urban areas was nearly two-fifth of households. As for tap water,

Table 3.2: Percentage Distribution of Households Served by Principal Source of Drinking Water in Rural Areas of Poor and Rich States, January–June 1998

State	Tap	Tube well/hand pump	Well
Bihar	0.7	70.3	27.9
Orissa	2.9	53.2	33.7
UP	8.8	63.5	22.1
Assam	7.3	49.5	27.8
Maharashtra	41.1	24.4	29.8
Punjab	14.8	82.7	2.3
Haryana	31.1	49.9	19.1
Gujarat	46.6	31.7	16.1

Source: GoI–NSSO (1999), Appendix Table 9, pp. A114-A123.

Table 3.3: Percentage Distributions of Households by Principal Source of Drinking Water and Distance from Source, January–June 1998

Principal Source of Drinking Water	Percentage of Households with Principal Source				
	Within Dwelling	Outside Dwelling but within Premises	Outside Premises at Distance		
			<.2 km	0.2 to 1 km	>1 km
Rural					
Tap	19.1	22.0	55.9	2.7	0.2
Tube well/hand pump	14.9	19.3	59.8	5.7	0.2
Well	0.0	22.7	66.4	9.2	1.6
Tank/pond reserved for drinking	0.0	9.6	65.1	15.4	9.8
Other tank/pond	0.0	34.9	47.6	12.2	5.2
River/canal/lake	0.0	0.0	57.6	38.8	3.7
Spring	0.0	0.0	39.2	28.2	32.6
All	11.0	20.1	60.4	7.1	1.3
Urban					
Tap	45.8	25.3	27.1	1.6	0.2
Tube well/hand pump	29.8	29.1	37.7	3.0	0.4
Well	0.0	45.2	48.9	5.6	0.2
Tank/pond reserved for drinking	0.0	10.1	46.9	35.7	7.2
Other tank/pond	0.0	6.7	56.1	31.9	5.2
River/canal/lake	0.0	0.0	54.5	45.4	0.1
Spring	0.0	0.0	92.5	7.3	0.2
All	38.6	27.1	31.5	2.4	0.4

Source: GoI–NSSO (1999), Table 3, p. 24.

19 per cent in rural areas and 46 per cent in urban areas had taps within the dwelling.

The results of the national Census of 2001 reveal that 28.7 per cent of rural households could get water supply within premises, 51.8 per cent near premises and 19.5 per cent away from their premises; the corresponding percentages for urban households were 39.0, 44.3 and 16.7, respectively. Table 3.4 gives Census 2001 results pertaining to percentage distribution of households by source of drinking water and their location. For rural households, hand pump is the most important source while for urban households the dominant source is tap. As for tap, about half of urban households had this source within their premises, but in rural areas less than one-tenth of households had this source within their premises.

As for the quality of drinking water, 85 per cent of rural households and 91 per cent of urban households reported that the principal source was of satisfactory quality (see Table 3.5). Tap and spring sources had the highest quality ratings. Common property water resources such as tank/pond and river/canal/lake had relatively poor ratings. Four decades back these were the principal sources of water for rural households. Their water quality has deteriorated over time.

The NSSO (GoI, 1999) also gives information about the sufficiency of drinking water available from different sources during different months and supplementary sources of water. Only 19 per cent of rural households and 65 per cent of urban households had bathrooms. Three out of ten rural households and one out of seven urban households had to avail facilities outside their premises for bathing (see Table 3.6).

According to the same source, 82.5 per cent of rural households and 25.5 per cent of urban households had no latrines. Of the households having latrine, the principal type is one with septic tank. Only 0.8 per cent of rural latrines and 22.5 per cent of urban latrines were connected to sewerage systems. Some 78 per cent of rural households and 26.3 per cent of urban households had no latrine (see Table 3.7).

The role of the local authorities in the removal of household garbage is also dismal. According to the NSSO (GoI, 1999, p. A166), the percentages of rural households expressing concerns about the problems of flies, mosquitoes and foul odour were 68.5, 84.0 and

Table 3.4: Percentage Distribution of Households by Source of Drinking Water and its Location, 2001

Source	Within Premises	Near Premises	Away	All
Rural				
Tap	33.5	23.6	12.5	24.3
Hand pump	42.6	46.7	34.8	43.2
Tube well	4.0	5.7	8.4	5.7
Well	19.2	20.3	31.7	22.2
Tank/pond/lake	0.6	1.1	2.7	1.3
River/canal	0.0	1.1	3.9	1.3
Spring	0.0	0.8	2.8	0.9
Any other	0.2	0.7	3.1	1.0
	100.0	100.0	100.0	100.0
Urban				
Tap	76.0	59.7	41.7	68.7
Hand pump	12.6	23.3	22.3	16.2
Tube well	4.4	5.4	9.2	5.1
Well	6.7	8.1	14.0	7.7
Tank/pond/lake	0.1	0.5	1.4	0.3
River/canal	0.0	0.4	1.0	0.2
Spring	0.0	0.6	1.2	0.2
Any other	0.2	2.1	9.3	1.5
	100.0	100.0	100.0	100.0

Source: Registrar General of India (2003), Table H-8, Census of India, 2001.

Table 3.5: Percentage Distribution of Households with Specific Principal Source of Drinking Water by Quality of Drinking Water from that Source, January–June 1998

Source	Percentage Reporting Satisfactory Quality	
	Rural	Urban
Tap	90.3	92.6
Tube well/hand pump	85.3	86.1
Well	83.2	89.5
Tank/pond reserved for drinking	68.6	76.8
Other tank/pond	55.4	65.2
River/canal/lake	67.3	52.7
Spring	90.6	97.0
Tanker	89.3	89.8
Other	76.9	91.5
All	85.1	90.8

Source: GoI–NSSO (1999), Table 12, p. 34.

Table 3.6: Percentage Distribution of Households having Bathroom/Location of Bathing Facility

	Rural	Urban
Households with Bathroom	19.0	64.7
Households without bathroom		
Bathing facility within dwelling	17.3	14.1
Bathing facility outside dwelling but within premises	33.2	13.6
Bathing facility less than 0.2 km outside	23.7	6.2
Bathing facility 0.2 to 1.0 km outside	5.8	1.0
Bathing facility above 1.0 km outside	0.3	0.0
Households not reporting	0.6	0.4

Source: GoI–NSSO (1999), Tables 15 and 16, pp. 37-8.

Table 3.7: Percentage Distributions of Households by Type of Latrine Used

Type	Rural	Urban
(A) NSS, January–June 1998		
Service latrine	2.7	5.9
Septic tank	7.5	35.2
Power flush pit	2.9	8.4
Sewerage system	0.8	22.5
Other	3.5	2.5
No latrine	82.5	25.5
(B) Census 2001		
Pit latrine	10.3	14.6
Water closet	7.1	46.1
Other latrine	4.5	13.0
No latrine	78.0	26.3

Source: GoI–NSSO (1999), Table 18, p. 40; Registrar General of India (2003), Table H-10; Census of India, 2001.

36.0 respectively. They reported that these problems increased during the last five years. As far these problems are concerned, the conditions are almost the same in urban areas.

Functioning and Use

Statistics on coverage of households provided by state governments in respect of drinking water supply and community toilet facilities relate to installed capacity and not actual use. The Tenth Five Year

Plan (GoI, 2002) notes that 'more than 3.5 million hand pumps and over 1,00,000 piped water supply schemes have been installed in the country under the Rural Water Supply Programme. A majority of the schemes remain non-functional and many others become permanently defunct due to lack of proper maintenance and repair for want of funds' (p. 604). In Maharashtra, out of 1.4 million toilets built at a cost of Rs. 4.42 billion over the past few years, only 40 per cent are in use. 'Either they were built at an inconvenient place or thrust upon the village regardless of whether they were needed or not' (Vijapurkas, 2002). We get similar reports about women's and children's sanitary complexes built in rural areas and small towns. Either they are not in use or not in full use because of lack of water, electricity and poor maintenance or/and located in inconvenient places.

Sustainability

The financial sustainability of the public water supply and sanitation system is being threatened because of the high capital costs of creating capacities, high operation and maintenance (O&M) costs and poor cost recovery. UNDP–World Bank (1999) notes that during the period 1951 to 1997, total plan outlays for rural water (including very modest amounts for sanitation) were Rs. 202 billion, and for urban water (also including sanitation) about Rs. 136 billion. It reports that a joint review of water resources management by the Government of India and the Word Bank arrived at 'rough estimates of recurring expenditure and investment needs for water and sanitation separately. For water in rural areas, the annual requirement just for adequate O&M is estimated at Rs. 29 billion. The investment requirement is over Rs. 200 billion to rehabilitate and repair all existing schemes and fill in gaps where necessary, and an additional Rs. 450 billion to bring the whole rural population to the "full coverage" standard of 40 litres per capita per day within a distance of 1,600 meters' (p. 10). As against the estimated annual maintenance cost of Rs. 29 billion, the annual provision for this purpose is about Rs. 2.5 billion!

Cost recovery rates for 15 states in India in 1993–4 were estimated at 5.16 per cent for water supply and sanitation in the (non-merit) services sector and 7.13 for sewerage and sanitation in the merit goods sector (GoI, 1997). The fiscal position of both the central and state governments has been worsening. The World Bank (2003) estimates the combined central and state governments' revenue and fiscal deficits in 2002-3, as per cent of GDP, at 6.9 and 10.1 respectively. As the public debt-GDP ratio is now more than one, deficits of these orders are unsustainable.

As the Indian economy is being liberalized and globalized, with the public water supply and sanitation systems and being costly, inefficient and heavily dependent on public funds, and as the central and state governments are not in a position to raise adequate resources for this sector, there is a case for adopting a decentralized approach based on PPP, which can be cost-effective and financially sustainable. The arguments that drinking water and sanitation are merit goods and that major water sources are common property resources do not necessarily imply that government be the service provider. What is needed is an appropriate regulatory framework to ensure that the needs of poor are met at affordable prices and that the common property resources are managed in a sustainable manner.

PUBLIC–PRIVATE PARTNERSHIP

There is a strong case for a decentralized and participatory approach to planning, developing and managing rural water and sanitation projects.[1] By involving the beneficiaries from the planning stage to the utilization stage and using the technical and managerial expertise and resources in the private sector, the government can create an enabling environment for achieving the social goals.

A decentralized approach facilitates finding location-specific solutions to rural water and sanitation problems. On the supply side, natural resource endowments differ from region to region. Annual rainfall varies from 10 cm in western Rajasthan to more than 900 cm in Cherapunjee in Meghalaya. Some regions are rich in water resources while others are poor. In water resource-poor regions, water supply can be augmented by exploiting groundwater, transporting water from nearby areas, rainwater harvesting, erecting recharge structures, and recycling and reuse of water. The unit costs of sources vary from region to region. Users' preferences regarding source of water, type of access (individual or shared), and location within dwelling or away, and ability to pay vary from household to household. These supply side and demand side factors can be taken into consideration at the planning stage, if the decision making is done at the local level with the involvement of the beneficiaries.

A major weakness of the centralized supply-driven approach is poor utilization of the capacities already created. The outputs are measured in terms of capacities created and the funds are disbursed on the basis of the output targets. For example, in case of hand pumps or toilets, what is measured is the number created. Little attention is paid to the factors which retard the maintenance and utilization of the assets.[2] In government budgeting, new investments get high priority and maintenance of assets get low priority. In fact, maintenance expenditures come under the category non-plan/ non-development expenditures. As mentioned earlier, the budgetary provision for maintenance of rural water supply and sanitation works is roughly one-tenth of the funds required. As a result, some of the assets created become non-functional. If the local community is involved from the planning stage and is informed of the technology, and held accountable for management of the assets created, we can expect efficient utilization of the assets created.

Decentralized and participatory approach can be cost effective. According to the World Bank (2003), the ratio of average wages in the public and private sectors which was 1.92 in 1993–4 has increased to 2.33 in 1999–2000, with premiums for government staff ranging from 27 per cent for engineering technicians to 145 per cent for low-end service workers (pp. 36–7). Corruption and leakages are not uncommon. Rural communities can create and maintain some of the assets at lower costs because their opportunity costs of time are low.

Rural water committees and self-help groups (SHG) can improve cost recovery at low transaction costs than government agencies. They are in a better position to allocate water resources in periods of scarcity as they have better information about supply and demand, and also use the social capital, i.e. norms, trusts and network to reach voluntary and binding agreements.

Local community-based organizations possess comparative advantage over outsiders in managing common property and common-pool water resources and in arriving at location-specific solutions to manage collection, disposal and recycling of solid wastes. What is needed is the creation of an institutional structure and an incentive-penalty scheme to induce them to undertake the chores in a cooperative way.

Government has to play a major role in developing a water policy, designing regulatory structures, accessing and transferring cost-effective technologies, facilitating design and implementation of large projects covering many villages and towns, executing the National River Action Plan and the National Conservation Plan, providing hydro-geomorphologic information and groundwater prospects to local bodies and private individuals to identify sites for constructing recharge structures and borewells, giving subsidies to poor, and supporting schemes where external/spill over effects are large.[3]

The private sector and NGOs can play an important role in identifying the technical solutions, mobilizing resources, undertaking supply contracts/projects/delivery systems based on competitive bidding. They can undertake projects on build, own and operate; build, own, operate and transfer; or some other bases. Private sector may be able to achieve cost savings and minimize wastages but they must operate within a regulatory framework so that the social goals are met.

Financial Sustainability of a PPP

A coordinating agency is necessary to coordinate the functions of different actors in a PPP project by designing an appropriate institutional set-up specific to the needs of each programme, and framing rules and regulations which induce the participants to realize that via cooperation each participant group can be made better off than otherwise.

Cost effectiveness should be the major criterion in capacity creation. Capacity costs can be lowered using locally available resources, traditional technologies, skills locally available, and reducing the construction time. The construction of a toilet in a rural area by the government costs around Rs. 5,000, but we observe that many NGOs and SHGs are able to construct similar toilets at half the cost. The wage compensation for masons, plumbers and other skilled labour in rural areas are less than half of the amounts paid to similar categories of workers employed by government. Rural projects can also be supported by partly using funds available under food for work programmes, minimum needs programme and other programmes for poor.

There is ample scope for reducing O&M costs of the assets created by entrusting the work to NGOs and SHGs. The repair and maintenance costs, revenue collection costs and monitoring costs are about half of the public sector costs when local community undertakes the responsibility. For example, rural people are willing to undertake the responsibility of managing sanitary complexes on a consolidated monthly pay in the range of Rs. 900–1,200 in many villages.

We need an innovative mechanism for sharing capital and operating costs of rural water supply and sanitation projects. For a public utility located in a rich village or town, where all households have meters, one can fix a connection charge based on the annualized capital cost and water charge based on meter readings to cover O&M costs. If the opportunity cost of water varies in different seasons, seasonal tariff can be introduced.

In many villages, less than 50 per cent of households would be in a position to afford household connections for piped water supply. Even these households may not be in a position to pay the connection charge if it is fixed in such a manner as to cover the entire capital costs at the time of connection. For such households, the connection charge has to be set below the capital cost and the water charge above the unit O&M cost, so that over a period of time, say within five years, the capital cost of water supply attributable to them can be recovered, and thereafter they pay only the O&M cost in the form of water charge.

More than half of the rural households can afford access to water supply only on a shared basis via tap, hand pump, well, or tubewell located near their premises. Part of the capital costs to people below the poverty line can be met using funds under the Accelerated Rural Development Programme, Minimum Needs Programme, Sector Reforms Programmes, and so on. There is scope for realizing the remaining capital costs by asking the users to make contribution in the form of labour during the construction stage. The major difficulty lies in the collection of O&M costs in the form of user charges on a regular basis because their water use is not measured. Local NGOs and SHGs can play a vital role in deciding the user charges as they can gather information about the water use by the households and as they have the capacity to monitor water usage and collect the user charges.[4]

Pay and use principle is being applied in public toilets in towns and cities. In some rural sanitary complexes set up by village panchayats, people do pay around Rs. 20 per household per month for use of the facilities. If 60 households use this facility and pay Rs. 1,200 per month, it is sufficient to cover the salary of a sweeper at Rs. 900 per month and water and electricity charges of Rs. 300 per month.

UNDP–World Bank (1999) gives many anecdotal evidences of the willingness of the urban poor to pay at least part of the costs of water supply and sanitation services. At the national level, the 54th round NSS results show that three-fourth of the rural households are willing to contribute money and/or labour towards improvement of sanitation in their neighbourhood. But only two-third of the households are willing to pay if the improvement takes place at the village level (see Table 3.8).

It may be observed that in both cases, majority of the households prefer to make their contribution in the form of labour only. Hence, there is a scope for designing a total sanitation programme at the village level funded partly by government and partly by villagers.

Peoples' willingness to pay for water and sanitation services will increase if they are assured of dependable and safe drinking water and hygienic community toilets and other sanitation services at convenient locations. At present, well-to-do farmers incur private

Table 3.8: Percentages Distribution of Households Willing to Contribute Money and/or Labour towards Improvement of Sanitation in Their Neighbourhood/Village

Contribution	Own Neighbourhood	Own Village
Money and labour	16.2	15.3
Money only	6.6	5.8
Labour only	52.3	45.4
Neither	24.1	32.3
Not reporting	0.8	1.2
Total	100.0	100.0

Source: GoI–NSSO (1999), Table 23, p. A-167.

costs for creating own water supply arrangements by having well/ tubewell and also for purchase of water from private sources. Even poor people buy water for drinking purpose or/and spend time in waiting or getting water from distant sources.

TWO EXAMPLES OF PPP

PPP can be a panacea for solving drinking water and sanitation problems only if it is demand driven, assigns complementary roles for the partners based on their capabilities, and finds solutions for market failures and government failures by designing institutions and regulatory structures to achieve economic sustainability. We illustrate issues in the design and execution of PPP projects with two examples.

Tirupur Water and Sanitation Project

Tirupur in the Coimbatore district of Tamil Nadu is a hosiery town. It is acclaimed as a model of decentralized and self-generating industrial development based largely on private initiative. The export of hosiery items increased from less than Rs. 100 million in 1984 to Rs. 20.72 billion in 1996. Rapid growth of bleaching and dyeing units and discharge of the untreated industrial effluents on to land and into water bodies deteriorated water quality to such a level that both groundwater and surface water were unfit for drinking, and in a few areas even for irrigation.

Public interest litigation culminated in an order in 1996 by the Green Bench of the Madras High Court for closure of bleaching and dyeing units which could not erect effluent treatment plants or become members of common effluent treatment plants by 1997. The bench also ordered the bleaching and dyeing units to pay compensation for the damages. The concentration of totally dissolved solids in groundwater exceeded 5,000 parts per milligram (ppm) while Tamil Nadu Pollution Control Board standard for treated water is 2,100 ppm and the desired concentration for domestic use is less than 500 ppm. As a result, both the industry and residents felt the need for safe and assured water supply. The Tamil Nadu Government was concerned about the possible loss of exports (of the order of

Rs. 40 billion) and the consequential losses in output, employment and incomes in Tirupur area.

The Tamil Nadu Government, Infrastructure Leasing and Financial Services (IL&FS) and Tirupur Exporters Association (TEA) took the initiative in establishing New Tirupur Area Development Corporation Limited (NTADCL), a special purpose vehicle, registered under the Companies Act 1956, in February 1995 to solve the water problem (see Box 3.1).

The specific services NTADCL include: (a) 20.63 million litres per day (mld) of treated piped water supply for domestic consumption to 5 wayside unions, 15 village panchayats, and 3 town panchayats; (b) treated piped water supply for domestic consumption to Tirupur

Box 3.1: Tirupur Water and Sanitation Project

This is the first PPP project in the water and sanitation sector in India. Tirupur Municipality (TM) and the adjoining villages faced severe water problem because of pollution of groundwater and surface water due to the discharge of untreated effluents by bleaching and dyeing units in this area. Public concerns, court orders and the need for helping the textile units with export earnings of Rs. 40 billion, brought together the Tamil Nadu Government, the Tirupur Exporters Association and Infrastructure Leasing and Financial Services to find a permanent solution to meet the water needs of the industry and the households.

The cost of the project is Rs. 10.23 billion of which equity is Rs. 3.227 billion and debt is Rs. 7.003 billion. The funds are contributed by the sponsors, financial institutions, insurance companies, and even foreign agencies. The project is designed by the British firm Bechtel; The construction work is by three Indian firms: Mahindra & Mahindra, Hindustan Construction Corporation and Larsen & Toubro. The operation and maintenance work is entrusted jointly to a British and an Indian firm. A Special Purpose Vehicle is responsible for coordination of all the activities.

The project envisages supply of 185 mld of water of which 139 mld is for industry and 33 mld for domestic needs. Industry will be paying Rs. 45 per kl, TM Rs. 5 per kl and rural villages Rs. 3.5 per kl. The project provides for sewerage system for TM and onsite sanitation facilities for slums within TM. The project is designed by Bechtel (UK). The contractors are operation and maintenance work is entrusted to United Utilities of UK and Mahindra & Mahindra.

Municipality (TM) to the tune of 12.5 mld; (c) 129 mld of treated water supply to dyeing and bleaching units within Tirupur Local Planning Area; (d) sewerage system for TM ; and (e) on-site sanitation facilities for slums within TM. The total water requirement is envisaged at 185 mld initially and it may increase to 250 mld. The project aims at building a 55 km long pipeline from River Cauvery, developing water pumping stations, a distribution network of about 350 km, and raw water and sewage treatment plant.

The cost of the project is Rs. 10.23 billion, of which equity is Rs. 3.227 billion (31.54 per cent) and senior debt and subordinate debt are Rs. 7.003 billion (69.36 per cent). The contributions of different institutions to equity and debt are given in Table 3.9. It may be observed that the three partners contribute Rs. 1.527 billion, which is 47.32 per cent of the equity. Of the total debt capital of Rs. 7.003 billion, two promoters IL&FS and TEA are responsible for raising Rs. 2.665 billion (38.1 per cent of debt), financial institutions and insurance companies Rs. 1.900 billion (27.1 per cent of debt) and the balance amount of Rs. 2.438 billion (34.8 per cent of debt) by commercial banks.

The proposed tariffs per kl of water are as follows:

Industries	Rs. 45.00
Tirupur Municipality	Rs. 5.00
Rural villages	Rs. 3.50

The above-mentioned rates are subject to escalation as per accepted formula. Water supply to industries will be available by April 2005 and water supply and sewer systems to TM will be available by October 2005.

It may be observed that industry alone would generate 97.7 per cent of the expected revenue of Rs. 21.68 billion while it is likely to use only 79.6 per cent of the water consumption. TM and the rural villages would get 20.4 per cent of the water supply but their contribution to revenue will be only 2.3 per cent. Hence, the domestic consumers will be cross-subsidized by the industry.

Even in 1999, the bleaching and dyeing units were buying untreated water at the rate of Rs. 30 per kl. The units with individual treatment and reverse osmosis (RO) plants were spending between Rs. 39 and 52 per kl on effluent treatment. Common effluent treatment plants

Table 3.9: Tirupur Water and Sanitation Project: Financing Plan

Sl. No.	Investor	Rs. crore
Equity Holders		
1	TWIC (Holding company of GoTN and IL&FS)	105.0
2	AIDEC Fund (Mauritius)	90.0
3	Wilbur Smith/Mahindra & Mahindra/United Utilities Consortium	45.0
4	Life Insurance Corporation	20.0
5	General Insurance Corporation	15.0
6	Tirupur Exporters Association	10.0
7	Others (Underwritten by TWICL)	37.7
	Total	322.7
Senior Lenders		
1	Industrial Development Bank of India	75.0
2	Small Industries Development Bank of India	60.0
3	Life Insurance Corporation	40.0
4	Central Bank of India	30.0
5	IL&FS (USAID Line of Credit)	90.0
6	IL&FS (Others)	90.0
7	Indian Overseas Bank	25.0
8	State Bank of India	50.0
9	Punjab National Bank	15.0
10	State Bank of Hyderabad	10.0
11	Bank of Baroda	20.0
12	General Insurance Corporation	15.0
13	State Bank of Patiala	10.0
14	Bank of India	10.0
15	Canara Bank	48.8
16	Oriental Bank of Commerce	25.0
	Total	613.8
Subordinate Debt		
1	IL&FS	66.5
2	Tirupur Exporters Association	20.0
	Total	86.5

Note: 1 crore is 10 million.

with RO plants were spending between Rs. 23 and 29 per kl on effluent treatment (Sankar, 2001). They could recycle about 70 per cent of the treated waste water and save Rs. 21 per kl. The expected effluent treatment cost when the new water service is available will be lower than the present costs. The industry recognizes its obligations to help the nearby residents for the past environmental damage. Thus, there is no problem in sustaining the cross-subsidization.[5]

The Tirupur Water and Sanitation Project is the first water sector-related project developed under the PPP framework in India. A Special Purpose Vehicle has been set up to ensure coordination among different partners, stakeholders, financiers and beneficiary groups. For the project design, construction and management it relies on the private sector. The project was conceived in 1995 but the services are expected from 2005. The proposed tariff structure appears to be fair and affordable. An automatic tariff revision formula linked to input costs and quality of service along with an efficient revenue collection system can ensure financial sustainability of the project.

Community Action in Olavanna

Olavanna is located in Kozhikode district of Kerala. Three rivers flowing through Olavanna Panchayat area are saline. Other non-saline surface water bodies go dry in the summer months. The water scarcity forced people to walk long distances to get water for their daily needs. The water supply schemes of Kerala Water Authority (KWA) and Gram Panchayats (GP) did not meet the needs of the people. A retired school teacher took the initiative of collecting money from five neighbouring families to install a hand pump with an intake well. As this demonstration was a success, it triggered many small communities to find local solutions to meet local needs. DFID (1999) gives information about how a rural community treats drinking water as an economic good (see Box 3.2).

About 50 households who wish to benefit from a piped water supply scheme in a village get together, draft their by-laws and register their cooperative society under the Cooperative Societies Act of 1860. The GP facilitates the process of forming a society. The society has an executive committee of between 7 and 11 members which runs the day-to-day affairs of the society. The general body which meets once a year elects the executive body for the next year, scrutinizes the accounts and discusses the annual report. There are about 26 such societies now.

A piped water supply scheme consists of an intake well, pump set, overhead tank and distribution system. The location of the well is arrived at by consensus. Land is purchased for the open well and the overhead storage tank. Local technicians construct the well and the storage tank and lay the pipelines. The construction work is

Box 3.2: Olavanna Community Water Project

Rural households in Olavanna, concerned about saline water in nearby rivers, non-availability of surface water during summer months, and erratic and inadequate supply of water from public schemes, found a local solution to meet a local need. Those households which desire piped water supply join together and establish a cooperative society, an institution for planning, development and management of the water supply system. The scheme consists of an intake well, pump set, overhead tank and a distribution system. Local technicians undertake the construction and complete the work between two and four months.

Each member pays a membership fee between Rs. 4,500 and 12,500 depending upon the cost of individual scheme. Water supply is metered. Every household is allowed 400 litres per day. During summer, water supply is reduced by mutual consent. The beneficiaries pay all the O&M and capital costs. Penalties are imposed for joining the project after its commencement and for delayed monthly payments. Poor households which want to become members can pay the membership fee in instalments. The schemes are functioning on a self-sustaining basis. The Gram Panchayat (GP) is playing the role of a facilitator.

done within two to four months. The supply of the water is metered. Every household is allowed 400 litres per day. Water is available 24 hours a day, except in the summer months when the supply is reduced by mutual agreement. Self-regulation is the preferred mode of regulation.

Membership fees varies from Rs. 4,500 to 12,500 per household depending upon the costs of individual schemes. Households desiring to join the scheme after it has been commenced have to pay twice the initial amount. The membership fees cover capital costs of the project. The beneficiaries pay all the O&M costs. For excess consumption they pay a penalty at the rate of Rs. 20 per kl. Fines are imposed for delays in monthly payments. Poor families can pay their membership fees in instalments. They are given an opportunity to earn wages during the construction of the scheme and use these earning to partly pay for their cash contribution to the scheme's construction. There is no subsidy or cross-subsidy for the poor. Some poor families have not opted for the private piped water supply scheme. They depend on public water supply schemes run by GPs and KWA.

From a comparison of the private scheme with GP and KWA schemes, a DFID Note (1999) concludes that the private schemes are more cost-effective, recover 100 per cent capital and operating costs, and achieve user satisfaction. One drawback of the private schemes is that some poor households who cannot pay the membership fees (even in instalments) and O&M costs, are denied access to the piped water supply system.

CONCLUSION

The need for PPP in drinking water supply and sanitation schemes is being felt in India to overcome the problems of market failures and government failures. The government has to fulfill its obligations in ensuring access to merit goods such as drinking water and sanitation services to all people, especially the poor. Association of the private sector is desired to get technical know-how, financial resources and management skills. Stakeholders' association is desired to ascertain users' preferences and demands, to reduce O&M costs of the schemes, and to ensure financial sustainability.

We considered two examples of PPP. The Tirupur Water and Sanitation Project costs more than Rs. 10 billion. The sponsors include the state government, the industry association and a leading infrastructure financing institution. The required finance comes from different sources—the sponsors, financial institutions, banks and even foreign sources. The project adopts a corporate management style, gets the services of international consultants and leading domestic construction companies. The project aims at meeting the water needs of the industry and residents in and around Tirupur town and sanitation needs of Tirupur Municipality. In view of the large number of agencies involved, a Special Purpose Vehicle has been set up. Even then the project would take 10 years for completion. The proposed tariff structure envisages cross-subsidization of domestic consumers by industry. It is not clear how the municipality and the panchayats will prescribe the tariffs and ensure payments to the suppliers.

The Olavanna water supply PPP is an example of finding a local solution to a local problem. The local government's role is only that of a facilitator. There is no dependence on external support for technology, construction or finance. It is a voluntary cooperative solution based on a participatory democracy process. It has a few incentive-penalty schemes to ensure prompt collection of membership fees and water charges, ration water in periods of scarcity and features to attract the poor. This scheme is cost-effective because of its use of local resources and skills and voluntary services provided by the beneficiaries. Being a private scheme, it does not aim at achieving the goal of providing water at affordable prices to the poor. The social goal of full coverage can be met if government bears part of the capital costs attributable to the poor, and the poor are given access to water on a shared basis via public taps with nominal monthly payments.

NOTES

* I am grateful to Meine Pieter van Dijk and Christine Sijbesma for comments and suggestions on the draft paper presented at the IDPAD Water Seminar in Delft on 13 May 2003, and to Sameer Vyas for providing information about Tirupur Water and Sanitation Project.

1. The Tenth Five Year Plan urges the need for decentralization of rural water supply. The Sector Reform Programme for Rural Water Supply and Sanitation introduced in March 1999 incorporates institutionalization of community participation through capital cost sharing and shouldering of full responsibilities for operation and maintenance.
2. The 'last mile' problem arises in the supply of many public utility services. When consumers are physically connected to service providers, as in electricity, telephone and water connections, the service providers can monitor the status and the consumers can communicate to the service providers about their supply problems. When the service is provided on a shared basis, as in the case of public tap or well, monitoring the service quality is difficult. A few state governments now encourage receipts of complaints about non-functioning of rural utility assets through the electronic media.
3. Rajiv Gandhi National Drinking Water Technology Mission initiated by the Ministry of Rural Development, Government of India, in 1987 enabled preparation of hydro-geomorphologic maps for locating sources of groundwater and identification of suitable points to build recharge structures in five states.
4. A lump sum monthly charge is easy to administer but it gives no incentive for the supplier to improve service quality and for the user to conserve the scarce resource.

5. According to Faulhaber (1975), a price is subsidy-free for a user if it lies between the incremental and standalone costs for that user. If the price charged exceeds the standalone cost, the user has an incentive to seek supply from an alternative source.

REFERENCES

DFID (Water Supply and Sanitation Programme), 'Villagers Treat Water as an Economic Good', Olavanna, Kerala, India, http://www.wsp.org/pdfs/sa_olavanna, 1999.

Faulhaber, G., 'Cross Subsidization: Pricing in Public Enterprises, *American Economic Review,* 65, 1975, pp. 966–77.

Government of India, 'Government Subsidies in India', Discussion Paper, New Delhi: Ministry of Finance, 1997.

———, 'Drinking Water, Sanitation, Hygiene in India', NSS 54th Round, January–June 1998, Report no. 449, New Delhi: National Sample Survey Organization, 1999.

———, *Tenth Five Year Plan 2002-07,* New Delhi: Planning Commission. http://planningcommission.nic.in/plans/planrel/fiveyr/10th/default.htm, 2002.

Registrar General of India, Table H-8, Census of India 2001, http://www.censusindia.net/2001, 2003.

Sankar, U., *Economic Analysis of Environmental Problems in Tanneries and Textile Bleaching and Dyeing Units and Suggestions for Policy Action,* New Delhi: Allied Publishers, 2001.

Vijapurkas, Mahesh, 'Budgetary Allocation for People-driven Scheme', *The Hindu* (Chennai), 17 March 2002.

UNDP-World Bank, 'Water for India's Poor: Who Pays the Price for Broken Promises?' New Delhi: Water Sanitation Programme South Asian Region, http://www.wsp.org/pdfs/sa_indiapoor.pdf, 1999.

World Bank, 'India Sustaining Reform, Reducing Poverty', New Delhi: Oxford University Press, 2003.

CHAPTER 4

Drinking Water and Sanitation in India: Need for Demand Management Structures

V. RATNA REDDY AND S. MAHENDRA DEV

INTRODUCTION

The scale of social consumption (comprising education, health services, drinking water, sanitation, and hygiene) and its distribution plays a vital role in human capital development. The extent of availability of social consumption items is governed by resource allocation and plan priorities. Distribution of social consumption influences inequalities in physical and human capital. The importance of drinking water and sanitation among these items cannot be over-emphasized.[1] Given the biological necessity of water for life, its availability, quality as well as quantity play a crucial role in human life irrespective of the socio-economic attributes. Historically, water has been a prerequisite for human prosperity and development. Besides, water stress also leads to environmental (micro) degradation. The majority of Third World countries are located in water scarce areas characterized by dry and drought-prone regions. Incidentally, these countries also fall in the bracket of large populations growing at high rates. Together, they make the adverse relationship between water scarcity and demographic pressure imminent. The situation of the Third World countries in this regard is quite precarious as their water use levels, though low on per capita basis, are very close to their ultimate water resource potential (Falkenmark, 1997). The fast exploding populations in these countries accentuate the impending threat to life from such trends.

Sanitation is closely linked with the availability of water. Together they determine the quality of life. Often scarcity of water results in low sanitation levels. On the other hand, poor sanitation leads to deterioration of potable water quality. A greater per capita usage of water demands more sanitation and sewerage facilities. Due to this intricate relation between water and sanitation, these problems need to be addressed in an integrated fashion. Besides, lack of awareness arising out of low literacy and neglect of gender needs are other important reasons for the poor sanitation levels in most developing countries. For instance, in India sanitation conditions are very poor in most regions/states irrespective of the availability of water. There is wide rural-urban divide in terms of access and availability of sanitation facilities in India. While lack of awareness and low priority are the main reasons for the poor amenities in rural areas, lack of proper urban planning is the main cause in urban areas.

Drinking water and sanitation have always been the priority of social consumption items in India. In order to meet the growing demand for these basic amenities, the Seventh Five Year Plan aimed at providing safe drinking water to all sections of the population. Even a decade after the Seventh Plan the objective remains unfulfilled. This paper looks at the status of drinking water and sanitation in India on the basis of the latest National Sample Survey data. Further, the paper examines the distribution of benefits from the investments in and subsidies on these basic amenities and suggests some strategies for improving the drinking water and sanitation situation in India. It is argued that the situation as far as providing safe drinking water is concerned is deteriorating and calls for steps towards demand management. The 54th round of the National Sample Survey conducted in 1998 along with earlier rounds brings out clearly the trends in providing drinking water and sanitation in the country.

This chapter is organized in six sections. The following section presents the status of drinking water and sanitation across the states of India. Section three discusses the financial allocations to water supply and sanitation while section four presents a case study on private initiatives in water supply. Section five examines the various aspects of residential water demand management based on the review of existing studies. And the last section makes some concluding remarks.

STATUS OF DRINKING WATER SUPPLY

Piped water is supposed to be the most reliable, safest and easiest source of drinking water available in the country. Hand pumps and tubewells are more labour and capital intensive respectively, though they are relatively safe. Access to piped water declined during the 1990s in general and in urban areas in particular. In urban areas it declined from 72.1 per cent to 70.1 per cent. In rural areas, access to piped water improved between 1988 and 1993 and declined marginally between 1993 and 1998 from 18.9 per cent to 18.7 per cent (Table 4.1). The second best sources, tubewells and hand pumps, are found to be compensating for this decline. Dependence on tubewells and hand pumps increased from 17.2 per cent in 1988 to 21.3 per cent in 1998 in urban areas and from 39.1 per cent 1988 to 50.1 per cent in 1998 in rural areas. Furthermore, the proportion of households going outside the house premises to fetch water gone up between 1993 and 1998 after showing a decline between 1988 and 1993, indicating an increase in time and energy spent on fetching water. Together the data indicate the declining quality of social consumption in terms of availability of piped water and the efforts involved in fetching it.

As per the 1998 estimates, 14.9 per cent of the urban households and 13 per cent of the rural households suffer from an insufficient supply of drinking water. Of these, 23.8 per cent of the rural households and 17.2 per cent of the urban households do not take any measures to compensate this scarcity, either by borrowing or buying. That is, at the aggregate level about 3 per cent of the population manages with an inadequate supply of drinking water. The conditions are particularly precarious at the state level. The number of rural households reporting an insufficient supply of drinking water ranges from 30.4 per cent in Kerala to 3.7 per cent in

Table 4.1: Access to Piped Water in India (per cent of Households)

NSS Round/Year	Urban	Rural
1. 44th Round (1988)	72.1	15.5
2. 49th Round (1993)	70.4	18.9
3. 54th Round (1998)	70.1	18.7

Source: GoI, 1999.

Punjab. In the case of urban water the range is between 30.1 per cent in Andhra Pradesh and 1.8 per cent in Assam (Table 4.2).

Andhra Pradesh is the worst affected in terms of severity of the problem, i.e. 8 per cent of the population faces inadequate water supply in both rural and urban areas. Tamil Nadu, Orissa and Karnataka also indicate scarcity conditions above the national average. Interestingly, states like Rajasthan with severe water scarcity do not reveal any alarming conditions in terms of households reporting insufficiencies or managing with too little water. This may be due to the reason that people living in severe water shortage regions are accustomed to low consumption levels. Besides, more households in Rajasthan purchase water to overcome the shortage than in other states (Table 4.2).

Shortages are met mainly by using supplementary sources like tanks and ponds. In the majority of the states (9 out of 15), households depending on piped water report water shortages during a part of the year (Table 4.3). This indicates that piped water is losing its

Table 4.2: Proportion of Households Reporting a Lack of Drinking Water and Measures Taken

State	Rural	Urban	Purchase of Water		No measures Taken	
			Urban	Rural	Rural	Urban
Andhra Pradesh	22.1	30.1	2.1	0.44	8.0	8.0
Assam	7.8	1.8	0.0	0.0	3.0	0.0
Bihar	6	18.9	0.17	0.0	1.0	2.0
Gujarat	12.3	17.7	0.03	0.36	1.0	1.0
Haryana	18	23.4	0.0	0.81	0.5	3.0
Karnataka	16.2	17.5	0.31	0.40	4.0	4.0
Kerala	30.4	15.4	0.18	0.30	2.0	0.4
Madhya Pradesh	12.9	15.8	0.0	0.06	2.0	1.0
Maharastra	25.1	13.7	1.23	0.20	4.0	2.0
Orissa	15.9	10.4	1.72	0.15	6.0	5.0
Punjab	3.7	5.7	0.0	0.0	0.5	1.0
Rajasthan	9.1	15.9	4.03	1.33	1.0	1.0
Tamil Nadu	18.2	12.9	1.50	0.52	6.0	2.0
Uttar Pradesh	5	7.3	0.02	0.03	1.0	1.0
West Bengal	6.2	2.9	0.20	0.02	2.0	1.0
INDIA	13	14.9	0.86	0.22	3.0	3.0

Source: GoI, 1999.

Table 4.3: Proportion of Households Reporting Insufficiency of Drinking Water by Source

State	Rural				Urban			
	Tap	Tubewell	Well	Others	Tap	Tubewell	Well	Others
Andhra Pradesh	31	14.2	14.1	17.9	47.2	49.5	25.5	43.5
Assam	18.7	57.6	46.4	49.2	76.6	84.1	67.1	77.7
Bihar	77.7	46	18.4	38.3	64.6	70.4	26.5	58.2
Gujarat	18.7	21.2	20.1	41.5	81	48.8	50.5	78.7
Haryana	77.7	39.8	8.6	29.3	84.4	76.7	0	82.8
Karnataka	65.3	10.7	34.8	19	66.2	16.2	70.6	60.2
Kerala	25	66.3	59.8	56.5	81.4	50.8	65.8	71
Madhya Pradesh	28.4	8.3	16.2	13.7	63.6	49.8	31	59.1
Maharashtra	31.9	13.6	19.5	29.2	81.7	45.7	27.9	78.2
Orissa	59.8	6.9	20.5	11.3	68.5	17.4	52	45.7
Punjab	48.7	89.8	19.2	81.9	94.5	93.1	100	94
Rajasthan	20.8	10.6	6.2	17.2	92	26.5	19.3	81.4
Tamil Nadu	48	18.9	13.9	16.4	48.2	63.8	30.1	48.9
Uttar Pradesh	49.7	58.8	15.3	47.5	88.3	71.7	23	77.1
West Bengal	16.9	26.8	19.5	25.1	57.4	31.4	73	47.8

Source: GoI, 1999

status as the most assured supply of drinking water in the country. This is mainly due to the poor management of urban water supplies. As far as the quality of water is concerned, 15 per cent of the rural households and 9 per cent of the urban households complain about poor water quality, which ranges from 40 per cent in Assam to 4 per cent in Karnataka (with marginal differences between rural and urban). In reality, 27 per cent of the urban households process the water before drinking (using other than cloth filtering). The practice reflects a substantial awareness of, and concern about, the quality of drinking water and adds to the cost of water.

The distributional aspects of drinking water are a prime concern, as the current distribution is uneven across space and segments of the population. Biases or inequities in the distribution are often attributed to demographic pressure, natural factors like rainfall, and policy bias. Population–environment linkages are well recognized and documented at the global level. These linkages are dynamic and unstable. The overall picture at the global level indicates a direct relationship between population pressure and environmental degradation. As long as population size and density adversely affect environment, basic resources like water continue to be scarce commodities. These conclusions, generally accepted as received wisdom, reflect the present global scenario. Of late, a number of studies have questioned this orthodoxy by providing counter-evidence, especially regarding the linkages between population, poverty and the environment at the micro level (Tiffen et al., 1994; Mearns, 1994; Leach and Mearns, 1991; Vyas, 1991; Reddy, 1999c).

There is a clear pro-urban bias in the provision of tap water. Within the urban areas, the bias towards the rich is of serious concern.[2] The higher income households are using the major share of the subsidized tap water. In most of the urban areas, stand posts or hand pumps are provided for slum dwellers. The low per capita water supply through stand posts is often far below the prescribed norm and aggravates the already existing subhuman conditions in the slums. Hand pumps also involve drudgery. The situation during the summer months is appalling with serpentine queues for collecting water from stand posts. And the dwindling groundwater tables make life miserable for the hand pump users. This inequitable distribution of water is a sign of socially inefficient allocation and wastage of scarce resources. This aggravates the disparities in the standards of living between the poor and the well-off sections of the society.

STATUS OF SANITATION

More than 80 per cent of the rural and 25 per cent of the urban households do not have access to sanitation facilities (latrines), although between 1988 and 1998 access improved from 11 per cent to 17.5 per cent in rural and from 68.2 per cent to 74.5 per cent in urban areas. More than 50 per cent of the urban households share the facilities with others. Orissa, Madhya Pradesh and Uttar Pradesh are the worst affected (above 90 per cent), followed by Bihar, Karnataka, Andhra, Tamil Nadu, and other states, in the case of rural sanitation (Table 4.4).

With regard to the urban areas, Bihar and Madhya Pradesh are the worst affected (over 45 per cent) followed by Orissa, Tamil Nadu, Andhra, and others. The performance of Kerala and Assam is impressive. In Assam, 98 per cent of the urban population and 75 per cent of the rural population have access to sanitation facilities, while

Table 4.4: Proportion of Households Without Access to Sanitation Facilities

State	Rural	Urban
Andhra Pradesh	88.5	30.8
Assam	24.7	2.0
Bihar	89.4	45.3
Gujarat	79.9	21.1
Haryana	84.5	32.9
Karnataka	88.9	30.0
Kerala	23.1	5.1
Madhya Pradesh	94.5	45.2
Maharastra	85.8	15.8
Orissa	96.1	35.8
Punjab	67.9	14.8
Rajasthan	87.0	25.5
Tamil Nadu	88.5	32.5
Uttar Pradesh	90.6	28.2
West Bengal	76.1	15.2
INDIA	82.5	25.5

Source: GoI, 1999.

in Kerala the figures are 95 per cent and 77 per cent respectively. States like Bihar, Madhya Pradesh, Orissa and Uttar Pradesh are at the other extreme. These variations reflect the states' commitment to ensuring sanitation and hygiene.

Only 6 per cent of the rural and 29 per cent of the urban households have access to garbage disposal facilities (Table 4.5). The majority of the households indicated that during the last five years there has been an increase in the incidence of mosquitoes (63 per cent), flies (48 per cent) and foul odour (22 per cent); only some 7 per cent of the households reported a decline. The problem of mosquitoes is reflected in the re-occurrence of malaria. An increased

Table 4.5: Proportion of Households with Domestic Garbage Removal Arrangements in 1998

Sector	Local authority	Private arrangement among residents	Household member(s)	Other arrangements
Rural	0.7	1.8	94.2	3.2
Urban	13.7	11.9	71.2	3.2

Source: GoI, 1999.

incidence of mosquitoes seems to occur more in the urban than in the rural areas.

Checking the declining trends in the provision and use of basic amenities such as drinking water supplies and sanitation facilities needs immediate attention at the policy level, since these problems are more strident as they directly affect human well-being. The main reason behind this state of affairs is the declining efficiency in managing the resources. In the case of drinking water, distribution and transmission losses are estimated to be in the range of 40 to 50 per cent. This could be brought down to 15 per cent through appropriate investments. In the absence of these measures, cost-based pricing in the name of economic reforms (as happened in Andhra in the case of electricity) would be unfair to the consumers. Effective real expenditure per capita in these sectors is also declining.

FINANCIAL ALLOCATIONS TO DRINKING WATER SUPPLY AND SANITATION

It is clear from the above discussion that both drinking water and sanitation conditions are much below the required levels. Though the drinking water situation appears to be better in terms of coverage at the aggregate level, the situation at the regional level, especially in the drought prone regions, is severe. While the coverage is above 80 per cent at the all India level, the coverage is less than 50 per cent in a number of states in the year 2000 (Table 4.6).

The financial requirements for achieving full coverage of all the habitations are above Rs. 11,000 crores spread over a period of five years (Table 4.7). The targets have to be reached by the year 2003–4. But, if the previous expenditure on drinking water and sanitation is any indication, it is unlikely that the target will be achieved. The annual expenditure (centre and states) is more than Rs. 2,500 crores in constant prices (Table 4.8). Expenditure for 1998–99 and 1999–2000 alone stand at above Rs. 10,000 crores. During the same period the proportion of habitations fully covered increased by less than five percentage points (Table 4.6). This indicates that either the financial requirements are under-estimated or the efficiency of expenditure is low. While expenditure increased by 86 per cent over the last decade, the share of the Centre declined from 21.5 to 18.8 per cent (Table 4.8).

Table 4.6: Status of Coverage of Habitations in the Years 1999 and 2000

States/UTs	Habitations							
	Not Covered		Partially Covered		Fully Covered		Total	
	1999	2000	1999	2000	1999	2000	1999	2000
Andhra Pradesh	0	0	24,683	21,583	45,049 (64.6)	48,149 (69.0)	69,732	69,732
Arunachal Pradesh	590	440	1,227	1,084	2,474 (57.6)	2,774 (64.5)	4,298	4,298
Assam	3,871	1,623	25,530	24,318	41,268 (58.4)	44,728 (63.3)	70,669	70,669
Bihar	1,069	625	564	144	2,03,803 (99.2)	2,04,667 (99.6)	2,05,436	2,05,436
Goa	34	16	34	44	328 (82.8)	336 (84.8)	396	396
Gujarat	437	293	4,639	3,127	25,193 (83.2)	26,849 (88.7)	30,269	30,269
Haryana	32	12	576	276	6,137 (91.0)	6,457 (95.7)	6,745	6,745
Himachal Pradesh	3,750	2,738	13,592	12,961	28,025 (61.8)	29,668 (65.4)	45,367	45,367
Jammu & Kashmir	2,430	2,348	4,047	3,726	4,707 (42.1)	5,110 (45.7)	11,184	11,184
Karnataka	845	65	25,037	23,129	30,800 (54.3)	33,488 (59.1)	56,682	56,682
Kerala	880	842	6,921	6,927	1,962 (20.1)	1,994 (20.4)	9,763	9,753
Madhya Pradesh	3,563	1,967	17,709	8,726	1,38,586 (86.7)	1,49,175 (93.3)	1,59,868	1,59,868
Maharashtra	3,171	2,597	32,119	28,740	50,640 (58.9)	54,593 (63.5)	85,930	85,930
Manipur	77	74	510	469	2,204 (78.9)	2,248 (80.5)	2,791	2,791
Meghalaya	874	633	1,276	1,127	6,489 (75.1)	6,879 (79.6)	8,639	8,639
Mizoram	2	0	624	569	285 (31.3)	342 (37.5)	911	911
Nagaland	428	417	703	670	394 (25.8)	438 (28.7)	1,525	1,525
Orissa	1,978	448	4,660	1,469	1,07,461 (94.2)	1,12,182 (98.3)	1,14,099	1,14,099
Punjab	2,266	2,050	3,123	3,123	8,060 (59.9)	8,276 (61.5)	13,449	13,449
Rajasthan	10,076	7,864	32,789	28,843	51,081 (54.4)	57,239 (60.9)	93,946	93,946

(contd.)

Table 4.6 (contd.)

States/UTs	Habitations							
	Not Covered		Partially Covered		Fully Covered		Total	
	1999	2000	1999	2000	1999	2000	1999	2000
Sikkim	0	0	732	624	947 (56.4)	1,055 (62.8)	1,679	1,679
Tamil Nadu	0	0	17,002	11,207	49,629 (74.5)	55,424 (83.2)	66,631	66,631
Tripura	726	541	1,604	1,198	5,082 (68.6)	5,673 (76.5)	7,412	7,412
Uttar Pradesh	845	432	20,158	4,999	2,53,638 (92.4)	2,69,210 (98.0)	2,74,641	2,74,641
West Bengal	0	0	28,101	23,732	50,935 (64.4)	55,304 (69.9)	79,036	79,036
Andaman and Nicobar Islands	0	0	176	161	328 (65.1)	343 (68.1)	504	504
Dadra & Nagar Haveli	74	56	259	259	183 (35.5)	201 (38.9)	516	516
Daman & Diu	0	0	1	1	31 (96.9)	31 (96.9)	32	32
Delhi	0	0	0	0	219 (100)	219 (100)	219	219
Lakashadweep	0	0	10	10	0 (00)	0 (00)	10	10
Pondicherry	40	40	90	85	137 (51.3)	142 (53.2)	267	267
Chandigarh	0	0	0	0	18 (100)	18 (100)	18	18
Total	38,065	26,121	2,68,496	2,13,331	11,16,103 (78.5)	11,83,212 (83.2)	14,22,664	14,22,664

Source: GoI, 1999.

Table 4.7: Year-wise Financial Requirement for Meeting the Demand

(Rs. in crores)

States/UTs	Year-wise Break-up					
	1999-2000	2000-1	2001-2	2002-3	2003-4	Total
Andhra Pradesh	91.43	220.00	265.00	300.00	365.00	1241.43
Arunachal Pradesh	24.76	12.40	12.40	12.40	12.45	74.41
Assam	31.92	16.61	15.19	16.14	15.07	94.93
Bihar	0	38.00	40.00	45.00	50.00	173.00
Goa	4.65	5.00	10.00	5.00	5.00	29.65
Gujarat	100.00	250.00	280.00	300.00	317.00	1247.00
Haryana	18.83	19.00	18.00	17.50	17.00	90.33
Himachal Pradesh	32.00	79.00	127.80	168.60	245.90	653.30
Jammu & Kashmir	64.00	70.00	75.00	80.00	86.00	375.00
Karnataka	150.00	400.00	400.00	400.00	462.00	1812.00
Kerala	23.59	59.77	102.06	121.55	141.97	448.94
Madhya Pradesh	94.44	110.66	125.00	55.90	0	386.00
Maharashtra	136.00	136.00	136.00	136.00	136.00	680.00
Manipur	6.11	12.00	13.00	13.40	13.69	58.20
Meghalaya	6.33	11.50	12.00	12.50	13.00	55.33
Mizoram	6.96	12.50	13.50	31.00	30.04	94.00
Nagaland	7.24	15.62	15.80	10.14	10.14	58.95
Orissa	97.92	61.59	7.08	7.08	7.08	180.74
Punjab	14.62	51.00	51.62	51.63	51.63	220.50
Rajasthan	109.00	110.00	110.00	110.00	275.00	714.00
Sikkim	4.60	4.60	4.60	4.60	4.60	23.00
Tamil Nadu	65.34	287.00	260.00	175.00	175.00	962.34
Tripura	14.70	26.55	20.21	16.42	10.61	88.49
Uttar Pradesh	125.59	161.50	180.45	191.25	191.25	850.04
West Bengal	70.00	155.00	155.00	225.00	249.00	854.00
Dadra & Nagar Haveli	0	3.00	2.00	2.00	1.00	8.00
Pondicherry	0.20	0.20	0.20	0.20	0.20	1.00
Total	1,300.24	2,32,850.4	2,451.91	2,508.31	2,885.63	11,474.59

Source: GoI, 1999.

The allocations to water and sanitation in the state budgets have more or less stagnated at about 7 per cent. The annual growth rates at the Central and state levels are highly fluctuating without any direction. This reflects the absence of any priority adhered to the sector. On the other hand, the situation calls for an increase in budget allocations on an increasing rate in order to meet the objective of drinking water and sanitation improvements. The present allocations are not even addressing the drinking water needs, let alone those for

Table 4.8: Financial Allocations to Water Supply and Sanitation

Year	Total (Central + states) expenditure (in Rs. crores – constant prices)	Share of central exp. to total expenditure	% of state budget expenditure*	% Change in state budget expenditure*	% Change in central budget expenditure*	
					Water Supply+	Sanitation
1991-2	2,913	21.5	7.2	–	39.1	-80.4
1992-3	2,685	15.9	6.9	0.4	-33.3	361.5
1993-4	3,098	19.9	7.6	10.8	45.7	45.6
1994-5	3,479	18.4	8.2	13.5	-0.1	70.5
1995-6	3,647	21.8	7.2	-3.7	26.5	-7.6
1996-7	3,980	18.7	7.5	15.4	-8.3	-7.0
1997-8	4,210	19.8	7.9	6.4	11.2	55.7
1998-9	4,712	19.3	8.1	12.5	13.1	-38.4
1999-2000	5,380	18.8	7.2	7.4	2.8	32.0

Notes: *Constant Prices 1993-4 = 100 (Annual Growth Rates). +Accelerated Drinking Water Supply Programme.

Source: Sharif et al., 2002.

sanitation. Many municipalities complain about lack of funds for drinking water supply and many more municipal and rural areas depend on private supplies at very high cost. This prompts us to look into alternatives to state-managed distribution. In the following section, we present a case study where private vendors provide piped water at a reasonable price to the consumers.

PRIVATE DISTRIBUTION OF DRINKING WATER: A CASE STUDY

In this section we discuss a case study where private people are involved in the distribution of piped water in a small municipality in Andhra Pradesh. While private water distribution through tankers in rural as well as urban areas is common, private supply of piped water is gaining acceptance in a number of urban and semi-urban areas. Such instances are spreading and observed in Karnataka, Rajasthan, and a few other states.

Macharla is a small town with a population of 50,000 located at the head reaches of the Nagarjunasagar Right Canal. The total water requirement of the town is estimated at 46 lakh litres per day (@ 92 litres per capita per day). However, the municipality is able to supply only 28 lakh litres per day (22 lakh litres through piped supplies plus 6 lakh litres through tankers). The shortage is more in per capita supplies, as the municipality covers 80 per cent of the population, although the shortage is 40 per cent in terms of water supplies. The main reason for the shortage is not lack of water as water is available from the canals, but a too small distribution network. It is proposed to construct two overhead tanks at a cost of Rs. 82 lakhs in order to cover the entire population. But the entire amount has to come from outside. Presently, income from the water charges to the users is Rs. 7 lakhs per year, while the cost of supply is Rs. 18 lakhs per year. If we include the capital costs, the supply cost will go up to Rs. 30 lakhs per year. As it is, the subsidy burden is huge even if we take only the recurring costs. The municipality charges Rs. 3,000 per house connection as part of installation charges and collects Rs. 60 per month (Rs. 720 per year) as user charges. No charges are collected from stand-post users.

Given the demand-supply gap in part of the locations and the demand for improved water supplies in some locations, some enterprising individuals speculated on the profitability in supplying drinking water to local households. After assessing the actual demand in terms of requirements and willingness and ability of the households to pay, they identified the most suitable localities. These are mainly those with above middle-income households. There was no reporting of any obstacles from the administration due to the need to expand the supply of water. Nevertheless, a nexus between the private suppliers and the department cannot be ruled out.

In order to meet the shortages, four private operators have started supplying water through pipelines. These operators have installed borewells in nearby locations and have laid distribution lines to the houses. Presently these private operators cover a population of about 10,000 people. They supply water for two hours a day, one hour in the morning and one hour in the evening. However, they do not treat the water. Apparently, there are no complaints from the users as they consider that the groundwater is pure. The fixed cost of private water supply includes the cost of drilling the bore and casing (Rs. 25,000) and a 15 HP motor (Rs. 33,000). Each pump can serve

2–4 thousand population (400–800 households). Their running costs include the electricity charges (about Rs. 3,000 per month) and operation and maintenance charges (about Rs. 1,500).

The pipelines were laid after collecting Rs. 1,500 per household. This is lower than the charges of municipality due to the shorter distances and also because people do not see the private supply as a permanent system and so do not want to pay more. The suppliers charge Rs. 100 per month per connection to the users, which is higher than the municipal tariff.

Even at the lowest level of coverage (400 households per pump), a private supplier collects about Rs. 40,000 as user charges and makes a clean profit of more than Rs. 30,000 per month after accounting for capital and working expenses.[3] The municipal authorities also appear to be happy about this, as the private people are shouldering the burden. This provides the rationale for joint efforts between the private and the public sectors. In principle, the public sector can improve the distribution and quality of supplies from complementary investments, whereas private parties can manage the distribution systems more efficiently and generate resources effectively through user charges. A co-production strategy may be better than leaving the supply entirely to private sector where consumers might get affected adversely due to monopoly power. However, the authorities are not keen to have a partnership and encourage the private sector to manage the water supplies.

STRATEGIES FOR MANAGING BASIC AMENITIES

Policy making towards resource management has hitherto been based on the philosophy of a supply-side management and has neglected the demand-side aspects. Demand management involves increasing the efficiency of water use by recycling, promotion of water saving technologies and pricing mechanisms. Although the supply of water is a major constraint in many cases, the major problem that leads to water shortages is the wastages through distributional and transmission losses and the inefficient distribution networks that presently exist. As the water wastage works out to be very expensive, investments in leak detection and leak proofing may prove to be more productive than investments in supply expansion. This, coupled with an efficient distribution network, would not only help increase the supplies, but also lead to more equitable distribution. The investment required for improving the supply network is substantial and so resource availability is the major constraint. In this context, demand management becomes critical for a sustainable management of the resource. Here we discuss the important demand management structures.

In spite of the rapidly increasing value of water resources, water demand functions are totally ignored in the major policy formulations. In most cases, projections of water demand are in terms of water requirements. The effects of the water prices and other variables on the future use of water are, therefore, not properly evaluated. The most important application of demand functions is in arriving at alternative projections of water use by systematically varying the factors that influence the demand for water. Moreover, the demand function provides a basis for evaluating whether specific investments in flow regulation and inter-basin transfers are justified (Thompson and Young, 1973).

Since they lack the scientific estimation of demand functions, most estimated projections are based on population projections and their normative requirements. However, the literature on water demand estimates for other countries, mostly developed, indicates that the quantity of the demanded water is significantly affected by the price of water and other socio-economic factors. Although the population size is the most significant determinant of residential water demand, there are other factors which play important roles in influencing the demand for water, such as the price of the water, variations in income levels, use of household appliances and size of households, the types of housing, the climate, and the socio-cultural background of the households. Broadly, these factors can be categorized into four groups, namely (i) economic, (ii) technological (iii) environmental, and (iv) socio-cultural. The price of water and the variation in income are the major factors falling under the economic category. Technological factors consist of water saving and water using appliances such as toilet flushes, washing machines, dishwashers, and so on. Environmental factors include average rainfall, temperature and humidity in the region, and the socio-cultural category includes the origin and nativity of the population and their water use habits.

Economic Factors

Economic factors have attracted more attention than any other factor in the analysis of residential water demand. In the literature, the price of water and per capita income of the population are considered to be the most important factors. Of these two, the discussion on price as a demand management variable has been the highlight of almost all the studies. In fact, an unsettled controversy still going on is regarding the specification of the price factor. Whether marginal price specification or average price specification is the most appropriate for estimating the water demand function is the bone of contention in this debate. Although the arguments in support of and against these variables are very interesting, we restrain ourselves from entering into this debate and concentrate on the price responsiveness of water demand.

Theoretically, the demand for any normal good is inversely related with its price, and positively related with individual income, *ceteris paribus*. All the studies testing these two hypotheses have revealed evidence supporting the theoretical propositions, although the magnitude of their estimates varies between the studies. As mentioned earlier, the available studies also differ in their specification of water demand function. There are some studies using average price alone and others using only marginal price (for a theoretical exposition on long-run marginal cost pricing, see Munasinghe, 1990), while some used both in order to test the specification bias. It is interesting to note that in all the cases the price elasticity turned out to be negative, although the elasticity of the average price appears to be larger compared to a marginal price specification. In the case of average price, the elasticity ranged from –0.1278 to –0.62 (Young, 1973; Gibbs, 1978; Foster and Beattie, 1981; Billings 1982; Jones and Morris, 1984; Cochran and Cotton, 1985; and Reddy, 1993a). On the other hand, the elasticity of marginal price variable ranged from –0.1216 to –0.6072 (Gibbs, 1978; Schefter and David, 1985; Foster and Beattie, 1981; Jones and Morris 1984; Chicone et al., 1986; and Chicoine and Ramamurthy, 1986). Thus, these estimates indicate that although demand for water is price inelastic (<1), its significance in all the cases reflects the importance of price as a demand management variable. The estimates show that a given percentage change in price results in a smaller percentage change in the quantity of water demanded. The price inelastic nature of the demand function for water is vindicated even in the context of India (Reddy, 1993a).

In most of the studies, income is used as proxy for other variables such as numbers of cars/vehicles in the household, the quality and type of the house, living in towns, and so on. These other variables are also expected to have a positive effect on water demand. The income elasticity as estimated in various studies ranged from 0.17 (Darr et al., 1975) to 0.51 (Gibbs, 1978). In the Indian case, the income elasticity turned out to be positive but not significant due to the measurement problems of the variable (Reddy, 1993a). These cases of positive elasticity indicate that as the income of a household increases, its demand for water will also increase. Thus, the price and income elasticity of water demand together imply that the average household considers water as a normal good. However, it may be noted that the demand for water is inelastic (in the majority of the cases the price and income elasticity hovered around 0.50), i.e. rise in price will result in a less than proportionate decrease in the water demand. It may be noted here that elasticity may vary across the income groups.

Technological Factors

When compared to economic variables, technological factors have hardly found a place in the demand function estimates. This is mainly due to the fact that most of the studies on water demand function estimates are based on secondary data, which may not provide household-wise information on water-using appliances. However, of late the discussions on residential water management are also focussing on these factors. It is argued that the spread of water-using appliances such as washing machines, dish washers and air coolers across the households and their expected future growth rates are vital for water demand forecasting (Whitford, 1972). It is further interesting to note that water-based toilets differ widely in their amounts of water use. For instance, a typical flush toilet in the United States (the biggest water user in the home) turns about 19 litres of water with drinking quality into waste each time it is flushed, against 9 litres in West Germany and 6 litres in Scandinavia (Table 4.9).

Table 4.9: Extent of Water Saving Through Various Techniques Available in the United States

Device	Water use	Per cent of saving over conventional methods
Toilets (litres/use)		
a. Conventional	19	0
b. Common low-flush	13	32
c. Wash down	4	79
d. Air assisted	2	89
Shower Heads (litres/minute)		
a. Conventional	19	0
b. Common low flow	11	42
c. Flow-limiting	7	63
d. Air-assisted	2	89
Cloth Washers (litres/use)		
a. Conventional	140	0
b. Wash recycle	100	17
c. Front loading	80	50
Faucets (Taps) (litres/minute)		
a. Conventional	12	0
b. Common low flow	10	17
c. Flow limiting	6	50

Source: Postel, 1985, p. 44.

It may be observed that water saving household appliances such as low flush toilets and water saving shower heads, cloth and dish washers can reduce water consumption by 50–70 per cent without affecting the quality of life adversely. In order to curtail this water wastage, a bill was introduced in 1985 in the California legislature proposing the installation of 5.7 litres capacity flush toilets mandatory for any new construction (Postel, 1985). This is a good indication for the developing world, which is at the early stages of this technology adoption, to make the appropriate policy changes.

In an earlier study Postel (1984) observed that water-conserving designs could enhance water saving from 10 per cent to 52 per cent, depending on the activity. Water conserving methods, if adopted, can reduce water use by 52 per cent in toilet flushing followed by washing clothes and dishes (27 per cent), and bathing (21 per cent). These new technologies not only conserve water but also prove cost efficient to the consumers. The investments in water saving appliances can pay themselves back within four years at most.

In recent years, Israel, Italy and the states of California, Michigan and New York have passed laws requiring the installation of various water-efficient appliances in new homes, apartments and offices (as quoted in Postel, 1984). Using this information we can estimate the extent of water saving in the urban areas. For this purpose we have used the item-wise water consumption data and estimated the requirements with new techniques. Simulations are worked out for different techniques in each category and presented in Table 4.10. The estimates indicate that water saving devices can drastically reduce consumption norms. In the Indian context, it is estimated that water productivity can be enhanced to the extent of 273 per cent through the adoption of various technologies currently available (Table 4.10). In fact, with the latest water saving devices water requirement norms can be fixed as low as 50 lpcd (litre per capita per day) as against the prevailing 135 lpcd. This results in the increase of water productivity to the tune of 273 per cent. On the whole, the extent of water saving

Table 4.10: Adoption of Technology and Urban Residential Water Requirement Norms

Item	Present Consumption[1] norm (lpcd)	With Various Advanced Water Saving Techniques[2]		
		Scenario		
		I	II	III
a. Drinking	5.00	5.00	5.00	5.00
b. Cooking	5.00	5.00	5.00	5.00
c. Bathing	55.00	31.90	20.35	6.05
d. Clothes washing	20.00	16.60	10.00	10.00
e. Utensils washing	10.00	10.00	10.00	10.00
f. House washing	10.00	10.00	10.00	10.00
g. Flushing of latrines, etc.	30.00	20.40	6.30	3.30
Total	135.00	98.40	66.65	49.35
		(73)	(49)	(37)

Notes: [1] Present consumption norms are fixed on the basis of conventional methods.

[2] Scenario I gives the requirement norm with (b) level technology as indicated in Table 4.9, Scenario II assumes (c) level technology and Scenario III assumes (d) level technologies.

Figures in brackets indicate the respective percentages to the present consumption norm.

Source: Data on present consumption norms have been obtained from Bride and Bridge, 1990: 79.

ranges from 27 per cent to 63 per cent depending on the type of technology adopted. Therefore, it is clear that through technology the quality of life can be maintained if not enhanced, even with low per capita water supplies.

Though the extent of water saving through improved devices is substantial, the adoption of these devices needs legislative and institutional support. Therefore, policy makers should bring in the necessary legislations in order to enforce the adoption. Most of these devices need little convincing at the consumer level as they are cost-effective and energy saving. Therefore, the stress should be at the manufacturing level, through discouraging the production of conventional devices and encouraging the modern devices. Furthermore, and as in the United States, the municipal authorities should consider this aspect while giving permission for new construction. Adoption of water-saving devices will also automatically take place when proper pricing policies are followed.

From the above it is evident that technological factors can play a major role in reducing water demand. Proper policies, legislations and institutions should foster these technical developments. For unless there are disincentives for not adopting these technologies, such as pricing, they may not be successful. Alternatively, their adoption should be made mandatory. Legislation can also help in streamlining the supply of technological devices in a desired fashion, i.e. permitting the manufacture of certain models. The third world countries, which have the advantage of being latecomers in this regard, can take advantage of these technologies through appropriate legislation.

Environmental Factors

In the literature, the analysis of environmental factors has only been cursory, although some of the studies have incorporated these variables in their demand functions. Rainfall, precipitation, temperature and evaporation are used as environmental factors in these studies. However, it may be noted that these variables either turned out to be insignificant or appeared with wrong signs in most of the studies and hence did not draw much attention. For instance, Young (1973) incorporated mean rainfall, temperature and evaporation in his study as environmental variables, but in the analysis only rainfall turned out to be significant with a negative sign. Similarly, in a district-wise study of Rajasthan, India, the per capita demand for water was observed to be lower in high rainfall districts and vice-versa (Reddy, 1993). These results indicate that the demand for water will be less in high rainfall regions or years, whereas higher temperatures and evapo-transpiration would enhance the demand for water. However, the reason for environmental variables not being significant in some of the studies is mainly attributed to the inability to separate the various classes of water users within the total water use (Cochran and Cotton, 1985). Therefore, these variables may play an important role in cross-section analysis across regions where climatic variations would be substantial (see, for instance, Foster and Beattie, 1981).

Socio-cultural Factors

Socio-cultural factors include household size, composition of the household, level of education, average age of the household heads, area of origin of the household, among others. However, most of the studies have used only size of the household as the social variable (see Gibbs, 1978; Foster and Beattie, 1981; Jones and Morris, 1984; Chicoine and Ramamurthy, 1986 and Reddy, 1993a). It is observed that household size influences the demand for water from two angles. On the one hand, it directly influences the total demand for water in the household, while on the other hand it reduces the per capita use. The latter is mainly due to the fact that given the size of the household and the facilities present such as bathrooms and various types of appliances, the general requirement of water for non-drinking purposes would not increase at the same rate as the number of persons in the household. Apart from household size, the other socio-cultural variables were analysed in a study of Israel (Darr et al., 1975). This study of eight towns in Israel incorporated age and education of the responding head of the household, and the cultural background, i.e. country of origin of the household, in the analysis of factors affecting the domestic demand for water. According to their estimates, education and age of the responding head of the household were observed to have affected the domestic water demand positively. For instance, when family size and income level are held constant, in each group (grouped according to the number of years of schooling) except for the small low income families, families in which the respondent has had at least 11 years of schooling consumed more water per capita than families in which the respondent has 10 or fewer years of schooling. However, the positive impact of education on per capita water consumption, though consistent, is not a universal phenomenon as it turned out significant in only three out of the eight towns studied and gender factors were not considered (it may make a difference on water use whether wife, husband or both are better educated). Similarly, the age factor turned out to be significant in 50 per cent of the cases.

For the cultural factor of country of origin, it was observed that, when family size and per capita income were held constant, Israeli-born respondents showed substantially less consumption when compared to households of Asian–African origin and those from Europe–America. In the higher income groups and at the same family size, European–American households consumed more while the consumption levels were more or less same for the other two groups. Among large families (four or more persons) with low incomes, there was little difference between the consumption of those of Israeli and of European–American origin whereas the Asian–Africans consumed substantially less. Thus, this analysis of cultural factor shows that people from perennially scarcity regions such as Israelis, Asians and Africans tend to still consume less water than those originating from North America and Europe. This may be due to the fact that in the scarcity zone people are forced to get accustomed to low levels of water consumption.

The preceding review brings out clearly that there are a number of social, economic, technological and environmental factors which influence water demand. Therefore, it is pertinent to keep these factors in view while analysing residential water demands. The broad issues emerging from the discussion are:

(i) Residential water is considered to be a normal good;
(ii) Its demand varies inversely with its price and directly with household income;
(iii) Price can be used as a demand management instrument as its elasticity, though significant, is on a low side and hence there is scope for increasing the price of water without reducing the consumption levels substantially. For estimating price elasticity volumetric charging of water is an essential condition.

For this, metering of water is essential, but is currently not practiced in the majority of India due to the cost factor. However, even from a cost angle pricing of water is important, at least to the level of covering the working expenses;

(iv) Less water-intensive technological adoptions can greatly reduce the demand for residential water without adversely affecting the quality of life;

(v) Family size has a negative impact on per capita demand for water and hence joint family structure and type of houses, which facilitate sharing may help in reducing the demand for water;

(vi) Other socio-cultural factors also play an important role in determining the demand for water though there is not yet enough evidence;

(vii) The demand for water will be lower in high rainfall and low temperatures zones.

Although these hypotheses are formulated mostly on the basis of the experience of the developed countries, they were also shown to be valid in the Indian context and are hence relevant for testing in other Third World countries.

In the context of developing countries such as India, the prime responsibility of developing and implementing these strategies lies with the government, as the onus of providing safe drinking water is taken by the State. Basically, the policy should address the issue of pricing in such a way that water is treated as an economic good. At the same time it should protect the vulnerable sections through cross subsidization. Thus, water should be regarded as a social good up to a threshold level (say 40 lpcd). Pricing along with other policy instruments such as legislation should be used to promote water-saving technologies. Taxing should be used to encourage or discourage the use of certain technologies. Even for encouraging private investments or fostering PPPs the government should provide a conducive policy environment.

CONCLUSIONS

Water resources planning and management has been a neglected area in India as well as other developing countries. As a result, the paucity of water is increasingly felt by all the sectors in most of these countries. The situation is more severe in the case of municipal water supplies. For instance, despite the best efforts of national and international organizations to provide basic amenities like drinking water and sanitation to all sections of the population, most of the developing countries, including India, failed to fulfill their objectives during the International Drinking Water and Sanitation Decade (1981–90). A decade later, the situation is only marginally better. The main reason behind this state of affairs is the philosophy of supply management hitherto followed by policy markers and their neglect of demand management structures.

Unless demand regulation is given importance in water resource planning and management, it will remain difficult to meet the demands of the increasing population, either in terms of water or food, seen the increasing water shortages and mounting financial constraints. Demand regulation includes the conservation of water, and enhancing the productivity of water through following appropriate pricing policies and adopting water-saving technologies with suitable legislation and supportive institutions. Often pricing policies are thwarted with an excuse of people's lack of willingness to pay for basic amenities. Contrary to this general belief, households are willing to pay substantially higher prices (double the present price) for improved water supplies (Reddy, 1996).

Therefore, willingness to pay is *not* a bottleneck for charging higher prices, as was also seen in our case study. In fact, it is the willingness to charge which is the main obstacle. Co-production strategies may facilitate better willingness to pay as well as charge. However, one should link the willingness to pay with the ability to pay. In contrast to the general assumptions that households are willing to pay about 5 per cent of their consumption towards water, in reality households' willingness to pay in most of the developing countries is less than 3 per cent of their consumption.

However, this willingness to pay may not reflect the ability of the households to pay, as the lower income group households are willing to pay a larger proportion of their household consumption towards water. Therefore, a blanket price policy may have an adverse impact on low-income households. Discriminatory pricing across income groups will be more appropriate. Nevertheless, studies showed that user changes could raise substantial amounts to meet more than the operation and maintenance costs even at low willingness to pay for drinking water (Reddy, 1996). The widely followed slab structure may be changed in such a way that lifeline supplies (say 40 lpcd) are provided at a lower price or even free of cost and then progressive pricing may be adopted using thin slabs (say 10,000 litres). The difference between lifeline supply price and the progressive price should be substantial.

Pricing of water on a cost basis is essential, because it not only helps in resource generation, but also results in efficient usage of water and discourages wastage of water. It is often observed that the decision makers, in the event of resource constraints, opt for permitting shortages and allocating water by non-price means of supply regulations when the existing capacities are on the verge of full utilization. Though this has become a norm in most of the developing countries, supply regulation is an unsatisfactory policy in the long run. Therefore, pricing policies should follow the marginal cost pricing. Marginal cost pricing requires that price should be equal to the short run marginal cost when capacity is less than fully utilized. But if demand increases and existing capacity becomes fully utilized, the price should be raised to ration existing capacity (Saunders and Warford, 1976). And when the capacity needs to be expanded, long run marginal costs, which include the cost of creating extra capacity, should be charged. The price would fall again once the capacity utilization is expanded.

Presently, only marginal amounts of water are being saved, recycled and reused. Experiences in other countries show the great potential of water saving devices, hence investments in this regard would be productive. Given the available range of water saving technologies at the international level, the extent of water saving ranges from 27 per cent to 63 per cent. However, these technologies need to be promoted with the help of appropriate policy instruments. Financial bottlenecks can no longer be given as an excuse, as the majority of the households (above 65 per cent) are willing to contribute to improve the conditions provided better services are ensured. Even otherwise, states like Kerala and Assam have shown the way to improve the conditions substantially provided there is policy commitment and political will. It is time to draw lessons from these states in order to improve the living conditions of the majority of the population.

Municipal waste management is another important area for improving sanitation conditions. Appropriate institutional arrangements need to be worked out to collect, recycle and dispose the waste. Some of the colonies already have arrangements (privately) to collect the household waste by payment (Rs. 15-20/month/HH). Such arrangements need to be strengthened and made more professional. Separation of garbage (organic, inorganic, glass, etc.) should be encouraged for easy and efficient recycling.

At the academic level, the area of residential water and sanitation management appears to be grossly under-researched in India. Very few systematic and scientific studies are available to guide the policy. Studies hardly focus on the effectiveness of the demand management structures on water demand though there are studies on willingness to pay for residential water. While lack of data is one reason, lack of demand for such studies among the policy makers is another. Therefore, we strongly argue that the research focus should shift towards demand management of this scarce and important resource. There appears also to be some scope for co-production strategies, although total privatization is not desirable in terms of equity and environmental concerns and ways are needed to ensure that private providers use part of their profits to serve the poor.

NOTES

1. The importance accorded to drinking water and sanitation is reflected very much in the proceedings of the Third World Water Forum in Kyoto, Japan.
2. The 54th round NSS does *not* provide information across income groups. However, the analysis based on the 42nd round NSS shows a clear bias in favour of the rich (Kundu, 1991; Reddy, 1996).
3. Even after including the tax on groundwater used for commercial purposes, i.e. Rs. 10,000 per year.

REFERENCES

Billings, Bruce R., 'Specification of Block Rate Price Variables in Demand Models', *Land Economics*, vol. 58, no. 3, August 1982.

Bride, G.S. and J.S. Bridge, *Water Supply and Sanitary Engineering*, New Delhi: Dhanpat Rai and Sons, 1990.

Chicoine, David L. and Ganapathi Ramamurthy, 'Evidence on the Specification of Price in the Study of Domestic Water Demand', *Land Economics*, vol. 62, no. 1, February 1986.

Chicoine, David L., Steren C. Deller and Ganapathi Ramamurthy, 'Water Demand Estimation under Block Rate Pricing: A Simultaneous Equation Approach', *Water Resources Research*, vol. 22, no. 6, 1986, pp. 859-63.

Cochran, Richard and Aurthur W. Cotton, 'Municipal Water Demand Study', Oklahoma City and Tulsa, Oklahoma, *Water Resources Research*, vol. 21, no. 7, 1985, pp. 941–3.

Darr, Peretz, Stephen L. Feldman and Charles S. Kamen, 'Socio-economic Factors Affecting Domestic Water Demand in Israel', *Water Resources Research*, vol. 11, no. 6, 1975, pp. 805–9.

Falkenmark, Malin, 'A Water Perspective on Population, Environment and Development', in Partha Dasgupta and Karl-Goran Maler (eds.), *The Environment and Emerging Development Issues*, vol. II, Oxford: Clarendon Press, 1997.

Foster, Jr. Henry S. and Bruce R. Beattie, 'Urban Residential Demand for Water in the United States: Reply', *Land Economics*, vol. 57, no. 2, May 1981.

Gibbs, C. Kenneth, 'Price Variable in Residential Water Demand Models', *Water Resources Research*, vol. 14, no. 1, February 1978.

Government of India, 'Drinking Water, Sanitation, Hygiene in India', NSS 54th Round, January-June 1998, Report no. 449, New Delhi: National Sample Survey Organization, 1999.

Jones, C. Vaughan and John R. Morris, 'Instrumental Price Estimates and Residential Water Demand', *Water Resources Research*, vol. 20, no. 2, 1984, pp. 197-202.

Kundu, A., 'Micro-environment in Urban Planning: Access of Poor to Water Supply and Sanitation', *Economic and Political Weekly*, vol. XXVI, no. 37, 14 September 1991.

Leach, Melissa and Robin Mearns, '*Poverty and Environment in Developing Countries: An Overview Study Report*', Brighton: Institute of Development Studies, University of Sussex, 1991.

Mearns, Robin, 'Institutional and Natural Resource Management: Access to and Control Over Woodfuel in East Africa', in Toy Bins (ed.), *People and Environment in Africa*, London: John Wiley, 1994.

Munasinghe, Mohan, 'The Pricing of Water Services in Developing Countries', *Natural Resources Forum*, vol. 14, no. 3, August 1990.

Postel, Sandra, 'Water: Rethinking Management in an Age of Scarcity', World Watch Paper No. 62. Washington, D.C.: Worldwatch Institute, 1984.

———, 'Conserving Water: The Untapped Alternative', World Water Paper no. 67, Washington, D.C.: Worldwatch Institute, 1985.

Reddy, V. Ratna, 'Demand for Water in Rajasthan: With Specific Reference to Urban Residential Water', Project Report, Jaipur: Institute of Development Studies, 1993a.

———, 'Beating the Big Dry', *Economic Times*, 6 September 1993b.

———, '*Urban Water Crisis: Rationale for Pricing*', Jaipur: Rawat Publishers, 1996.

———, 'Quenching the Thirst: Means and Costs in Fragile Environments', *Development and Change*, vol. 30, no. 1, January 1999b.

———, 'Pricing of Rural Drinking Water: A Study of Willingness and Ability to Pay in Western Rajasthan', *Journal of Social and Economic Development*, vol. 2, no. 1, January 1999a.

———, 'User Valuation of Renewable Natural Resources: User Perspective', *Economic and Political Weekly*, vol. XXXIV, no. 23, 5 June 1999b.

Saunders, Robert J. and Jeremy J. Warford, 'Village Water Supply: Economics and Policy in the Developing World', Baltimore and London: John Hopkins University Press, 1976.

Schefter, J.E. and E.L. David, 'Estimating Residential Water Demand under Multi-part Tariffs using Aggregate Data', *Land Economics*, vol. 61, no. 3, August 1985.

Sharif, A., Prabir Ghosh and S.K. Mondal, 'State-adjusted Public Expenditure on Social Sector and Poverty Alleviation Programmes', *Economic and Political Weekly*, vol. XXXVII, no. 8, 23 February 2002.

Thompson, Russell G. and H. Peyton Young, 'Forecasting Water Use for Policy Making: A Review', *Water Resources Research*, vol. 9, no. 4, August 1973.

Tiffen, M. et al., *More People, Less Erosion*, Chichester: John Wiley and Sons, 1994.

Vyas, V.S., 'Agrarian Structure, Environmental Concerns and Rural Poverty', Elmhurst Memorial Lecture, XXI International Conference of Agricultural Economists, Tokyo, Japan, 22 August 1991.

Whitford, Peter W., 'Residential Water Demand Forecasting', *Water Resources Research*, vol. 8, no. 4, August 1972.

Young, Robert A., 'Pricing Elasticity of Demand for Municipal Water: A Case Study of Tucson, Arizona', *Water Resources Research*, vol. 9, no. 4, August 1973.

CHAPTER 5

Water Sector Reform Policy and Operationalization: Experiences in Gujarat

K. PRATHAP REDDY

INTRODUCTION

Water is the very basis for the existence of human as well as all other forms of life. Access to safe water and sanitation is a critical socio-economic, environmental and in many cases a political issue, which determines the health of individuals and communities and the productivity of nations. Historically, drinking water in rural India was managed outside the government's sphere of influence or responsibility. Community managed open wells, private wells, tanks, and ponds were and continue to be the main source of rural drinking water supply. Government-installed wells and bore holes first appeared in early 1950s as part of the government's policy to meet basic needs of its people. Since then, the government's control over rural water supply has increased and the involvement of local people and communities has continuously decreased (World Bank, 1999).

The primary responsibility for providing drinking water and sanitation (WATSAN) in the country rests with the state governments. The Government of India mainly ensures that funds are provided in state budgets, and progressively larger allocations are made for water supply and sanitation in the various five-year plans. The first national WATSAN programme was launched in 1954, during the First Five-Year Plan, as part of the government's health plan. The state public health and engineering departments were strengthened in the three subsequent five-year plans (World Bank, 1999). During this fifteen-year period, rural water schemes were expanded to include small towns with populations less than 20,000, and priority was given to problem villages, where the scarcity of drinking water was deemed particularly severe.

Although the first four five-year plans made some progress, it was much below the desired level. Therefore, the Government of India introduced the Accelerated Rural Water Supply Programme (ARWSP) in 1972–3 to assist the states and union territories to accelerate the pace and coverage of drinking water supply. Through the ARWSP, the Government of India supplemented the efforts of the state governments by providing financial assistance and technical guidance. The significance of providing safe drinking water and sanitation as a basic minimum need was felt in the Fifth Five Year Plan (1974–9), which included rural water supply in its Minimum Needs Programme (MNP). The AWRSP was discontinued with the introduction of the MNP in 1974–5. However, AWRSP was reintroduced in 1977–8 when progress in supplying safe drinking water to identified problem villages had been poor. The entire programme was given a mission approach in 1986 with the National Drinking Water Mission (NDWM). It was renamed Rajiv Gandhi National Drinking Water Mission (RGNDWM) in 1991. The Government of India introduced yet another programme —Swajaldhara Programme—in November 2002 to give further impetus to the water sector reform efforts.

THIRSTY AND UNCLEAN VILLAGES

India has made tremendous progress due to government interventions and WATSAN sector reform efforts in rural water supply and sanitation sectors. The drinking water supply coverage of households in urban areas and habitations in rural areas increased from 77 per cent and 31 per cent in 1980 to 94 per cent and 80 per cent in 2000 respectively (Fig. 5.1). Another way of looking at it is that nearly 28,000 rural habitations did not have safe drinking water supply in 2000 in India.

The coverage of sanitation is still poor. It was as low as 27 per cent and 1 per cent in 1980 and increased to 76 per cent and 18 per cent in 2000 in the urban and rural areas respectively. That means that more than a million habitations in India did not have proper sanitation facilities even in 2000. This coverage is perhaps on the basis of the concept of sanitation limited to disposal of human excreta by

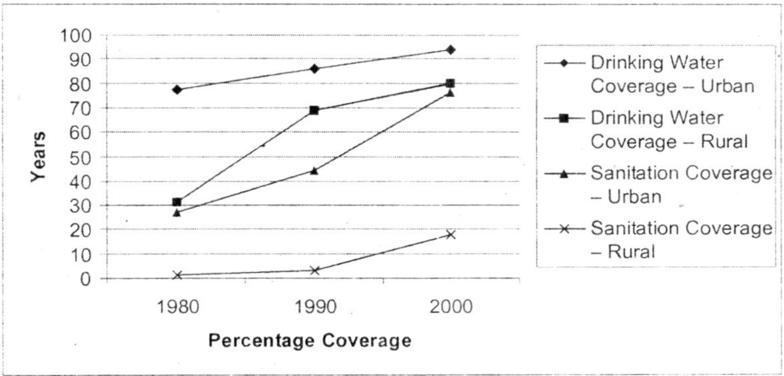

Source: WHO/UNICEF, 2003.

Fig. 5.1: Extent of Water Supply and Sanitation Coverage in India

cess pools, open ditches, pit latrines, and bucket system. However, if we use the more comprehensive concept of sanitation, which includes liquid and solid waste disposal, as well as personal, domestic, environmental and food hygiene, the coverage would be dismal.

The problem of poor coverage of drinking water supply is further compounded by the significant regional imbalances in the coverage and seasonal variations. Some states like Kerala, Punjab, West Bengal and some north-eastern states have a significantly lower coverage, while a few others, such as Tamil Nadu, Delhi and Haryana have done exceedingly well, as shown in Table 5.1.

The accuracy of the data is doubtful, however. For example, the webpage of the Comptroller and Auditor General of India gives the number of villages as 1,430,543 (GoI, 2002). Similarly, the coverage of rural habitations with safe drinking water is 86 per cent according to a presentation made by UNICEF in a state-level consultative workshop on 30 April 2003. For Gujarat, a coverage of more than 95 per cent rural habitations under rural drinking water supply is given. This is, however, not entirely correct. Many districts in northern Gujarat and Saurashtra are facing perennial drinking water problem, especially in summers.

Another issue of concern is that of sustainability. It is known that some of the water sources go dry after a few years or in summer, in both partially and fully covered villages, thereby making them problem villages. It should be remembered that no drinking water solution is

Table 5.1: Status of Drinking Water Supply in Rural Habitations (as on 28 January 2003)

Sl. No.	State/UTs	Percentage Coverage of Rural Habitations			Total
		NC	PC	FC	
1	Andhra Pradesh	0.00	19.85	80.15	69,732
2	Arunachal Pradesh	7.56	20.47	71.96	4,298
3	Assam*	0.62	24.88	74.49	70,669
4	Bihar	0.00	0.00	100.00	1,05,340
5	Chhattisgarh	0.00	0.00	100.00	50,379
6	Goa	2.02	10.10	87.88	396
7	Gujarat	0.17	4.72	95.12	30,269
8	Haryana	0.00	0.71	99.29	6,745
9	Himachal Pradesh	1.81	20.45	77.74	45,367
10	Jammu & Kashmir	15.28	31.97	52.74	11,184
11	Jharkhand	0.23	0.04	99.72	1,00,096
12	Karnataka	0.00	31.46	68.54	56,682
13	Kerala	8.01	70.46	21.53	9,763
14	Madhya Pradesh	0.00	0.00	100.00	1,09,489
15	Maharashtra	2.33	27.95	69.72	85,930
16	Manipur	0.14	6.56	93.30	2,791
17	Meghalaya	3.79	9.12	87.09	8,639
18	Mizoram	0.00	49.84	50.16	911
19	Nagaland	22.89	37.31	39.80	1,525
20	Orissa	0.00	0.00	100.00	1,14,099
21	Punjab	10.36	15.72	73.92	13,449
22	Rajasthan	5.99	2.68	91.32	93,946
23	Sikkim	0.00	17.27	82.73	1,679
24	Tamil Nadu	0.00	0.00	100.00	66,631
25	Tripura	1.25	0.27	98.48	7,412
26	Uttar Pradesh**	0.00	0.00	100.00	2,43,633
27	Uttaranchal	0.38	2.94	96.67	31,008
28	West Bengal	0.00	11.46	88.54	79,036
29	A & N Islands	0.00	24.01	75.99	504
30	D & N Haveli	5.81	46.71	47.48	516
31	Daman & Diu	0.00	0.00	100.00	32
32	Delhi	0.00	0.00	100.00	219
33	Lakshadweep	0.00	100.00	0.00	10
34	Pondicherry	14.98	26.22	58.80	267
35	Chandigarh	0.00	0.00	100.00	24
	Total	1.01	7.93	91.06	14,22,664

Notes: Not covered (< 10 lpcd); PC: Partially covered (10-40 lpcd); FC: Fully covered (> 40 lpcd); *114 habitations do not exist now; **125 habitations merged with urban areas.

Source: Government of India, 2003.

permanent; a solution lasts for a limited period—may be for 5, 10 or 20 years.

The quality of the water is another major problem. The Government of India appointed a Ground Water Sub-Group (Government of India, 1997), which found that (i) arsenic affects drinking water in 1,000 habitations in West Bengal; (ii) high fluoride affects nearly 28,000 habitations in Andhra Pradesh, Gujarat, Haryana, Karnataka, Punjab, Rajasthan, Tamil Nadu and Utter Pradesh; (iii) high iron levels affect nearly 58,000 habitations in the northern and eastern parts of India; and (iv) high salinity exists in Gujarat, Haryana, Karnataka, Punjab, Rajasthan and Tamil Nadu. According to a report in the *Indian Express* (27 April 2003), almost every household had at least one person suffering from kidney stone problem in most villages of Jamnagar district in coastal Gujarat, which is caused by excessive salinity.

Although the government figures show that the extent of coverage of rural habitations with safe drinking water is improving over the years, the per capita availability seems to be declining quite rapidly, suggesting a mammoth fresh water crisis. In 1951, the per capita availability of fresh water in India was 3,450 m^3 per year. In 1999, it stood at approximately 1,250 m^3 per capita per year and it will reduce to 760 m^3 in the year 2050 (Government of India, 1999). The per capita decline of water availability, however, does not necessarily contribute to water scarcity in the absolute sense. There are a few but distinct cases of community initiatives that have enabled people to survive the scarcity of water through collective action and prudent water management, even with very little water availability. The abundance of water also does not ensure that water will be available to everyone. History is replete with examples of famines and droughts that have more to do with man-made situations than nature failure.

THE INDIAN SECTOR REFORMS

The state governments were entrusted with the responsibility for rural water supply and sanitation programmes. Many state governments have created a separate department (Public Health and Engineering Department (PHED) or a board, such as the Gujarat Water Supply and Sewerage Board (GWSSB), for managing these programmes. The support of the Government of India was mainly to help state governments provide drinking water and sanitation facilities in problem villages (not covered and partially covered habitations) through AWRSP and MNP. The departments/boards designed and executed the water and sanitation systems/schemes and imposed them on the end-users. Demand preferences of the people were not taken into account while executing the schemes. As a result, water is today perceived by the rural public as a social right, to be provided free by the government, rather than as a scarce resource which must be managed locally as a socio-economic good in order to ensure its effective use. This supply-driven approach has led to the failure of a large number of water supply and sanitation systems/schemes due to poor operation and maintenance.

Now that substantial investments have been made in the sector and a huge infrastructure built up, it is paramount that the systems are made functional to a great degree and achieve sustainability. There is a general recognition that a transformation from a target-based supply-driven approach, which pays little attention to the actual practices and/or preferences of the end users, to a demand-based approach where users get the service they want and are willing to pay for, is urgently required. Implementation of a participatory demand-driven approach will ensure that the public obtain the level of service they desire and can afford to pay. Further, full cost recovery of operations and maintenance and replacement costs will ensure the financial viability and sustainability of the schemes.

The main principles underlying the WATSAN sector reforms identified and emphasized in the Eighth Five Year Plan are: (i) the delivery of water should be managed as a commodity in the same manner as any other resource; (ii) the delivery of water services should be based on the principle of effective demand and should correspond to the standard of service that users are willing to maintain, operate and finance; (iii) local bodies (i.e. the Panchayati Raj Institutions, or PRI) should be responsible for operating and maintaining the system installed; (iv) local bodies should be free to levy and raise appropriate user charges for drinking water and sanitation services, undertaking operations and maintenance if not further investment, and be self-sustaining; (v) the private sector should be encouraged to construct and maintain schemes to the maximum extent feasible; and (vi) appropriate links should be forged between water supply and environment sanitation. The pilot projects initiated by RGNDWS in 1997 and the Swajaldhara Programme launched in November 2002 are based on these principles.

Despite enhanced resources being directed to the development of the WATSAN sector and the recognition of the need for decentralized and participatory water management, there is still a limited understanding of the concept of 'community' amongst policy makers and development practitioners, providing for a more active role for local communities in the management of their water-related needs. Social mobilization is seen as promoting partnerships between different stakeholders and enhancing the delivery of resources and services towards sustainable water management. Yet, the essential condition for the success of such efforts is behavioural change at all the levels—from users to technical staff—and promoting/funding agencies. Otherwise the concepts of community participation and partnership will remain rhetoric, and the goals of providing access to safe water and sanitation, particularly to the millions of poor and marginalized communities, will not be achieved. Current initiatives in several states of India include the transfer of responsibilities from bureaucratic water supply agencies to local people's organizations. These provide development agencies with a key role in the WATSAN sector in India, and a platform for the demonstration and application of successful principles of community-managed water supply and sanitation interventions.

THE EMERGING INSTITUTIONAL AND POLICY ISSUES

The emerging issues presented in this paper are based on our work at IRMA and my understanding of the WATSAN sector reform efforts, mainly in Gujarat and to a limited extent in Andhra Pradesh and Kerala.

The main issue in the WATSAN sector is sustaining the supply of adequate quantity of quality drinking water, the demand for which is increasing due to population growth as well as demand for higher level of service. During the drought of 2000, for example, nearly 25 million people in 9,500 villages, 4 metros, and 79 towns in Gujarat were hit by drinking water scarcity (IRMA, 2001). The impact of subsequent droughts in Gujarat and in other parts of India is equally serious. Water scarcity and the emerging issues are discussed in the following pages.

Policy Formulation

The discourse on water is dominated by thinking of projected and perceived water scarcity. Once this paradigm is accepted, what follows is a discussion of a series of issues that pertain to practical solution of accepted principles, such as how to increase supply, by how much, and what technology to use. Connected with these is the political nature of policy formulation and implementation process, policy as contested by the different interest groups at all stages of its existence trying to shape it in particular ways. In the current discourse on politics of policy making for the water sector, there are two dominant paradigms. One of these places greater emphasis on technology and building infrastructure, and the other on stakeholders' participation. But, the discussion about how and in what way policy is formulated and evolved is generally missing. The need for stakeholders' participation in policy formulation is recognized and enlisted but their representation is highly questionable. Discourses on water politics among civil society organizations are also narrowly constructed. This formulation of discourse is largely concerned about commodification of water, and educating users to pay at least for Operation and Maintenance (O&M) of water and sanitation structures. The larger debate about reorientation of water-related departments are generally missing (Ballabh, 2003).

The policy of assuming increasing responsibility for the WATSAN sector by the government over the years has disempowered the users and the local institutions, relieving them of the need to take responsibility for their own needs. This is true not only in the WATSAN sector but in all the development efforts of government. There is a need to redefine the roles and responsibilities of various stakeholders —a paradigm shift towards people-centred approach, which needs acceptance of water as an economic resource. The shift is of a kind, not of a degree. The next section will discuss a model proposed by IRMA to the state government of Gujarat.

Water Rights

Effective management of water resources is closely linked with the structure of property right over water. In Gujarat and elsewhere in India, the legal rights over surface water such as rivers, lakes, ponds and tanks, are vested in the state, except for those which are under private ownership. The legal rights over groundwater resources are not clear. De facto, groundwater belongs to those who own the overlying piece of land, as per the British Common Law. This has led to indiscriminate exploitation of ground water, leading to serious water scarcity as well as quality problems (IRMA, 2001).

Equity Issues

The growing scarcity and ineffective institutional arrangements for capture, allocation and distribution compounds the growing water crisis and shortages. These crises are unlikely to be resolved by increasing the water supply. When requirement exceeds supply, the extra supply created is diverted to already well-off people. In the struggle for capture and control over scarce water, those left out are among the poorest of our society—the poor and marginal farmers, and domestic water users both in rural and urban areas. Equitable water distribution of scarce water among multiple users poses a major challenge. Mismanagement of water in the deficient areas is also quite common. The natural scarcity of water is thus aggravated by its use by a few. Confining the use of existing resources for higher consumptive practices thus artificially generates part of the water shortages. The current state policies promote high water-intensive crops and water-consuming and chemical-based industries, which not only consume lot of water but also create pollution. One of the major externality of the above is the adverse impact on availability of sufficient clean drinking water (Ballabh, 2003).

When water is scarce, it is the poor and the women who suffer the most—women with the drudgery of collecting water from far-off places, and the poor due to lack of access. Equity issues could be addressed if investments are made in communication and education for building awareness and capabilities in the local populations. The governance of water services to address the equity issues depends largely on the effectiveness of the institutional structure. But in

Gujarat, the agencies responsible for management of water lack the instruments—legal and economic—that can influence the desired changes in water use. As a result, these agencies are unable to decide on priority for water allocation, and have inability to control pollution, and resolve conflicts over water use.

Centralized Direction

Implementing agencies are operating under centrally sponsored programmes and centrally guided policies. The older ARWSP and MNP and the recently launched RGNDWS pilot projects and the Swajaldhara Programmes provide very detailed guidelines to be followed by the implementing agencies and thus limiting their flexibility. Moreover, the central guidelines disregard the local variations of territorial, topographical, hydrological, and socio-cultural aspects. A habitat dependent on cattle as main source of livelihood has a different need than one dependent on agriculture. Such centralized directions limit the search for more appropriate and low cost options for service delivery. Community participation is limited to providing the prescribed level of contribution, in kind or cash, in the implementation of these programmes. Though the guidelines suggest active involvement of local people, especially the women and weaker sections, it is more often breached than followed.

For example, the Gujarat Water Supply and Sanitation Board has a provision of about Rs. 585 for annual maintenance of hand pumps. But it also has a rule that the contract for the maintenance could be given based on competitive tenders. And everyone knows how the tendering system works. The women and the poor would hardly have a chance to get the contract for their own village hand pumps, if there is no intervention from an organization like SEWA. Is it necessary to insist on contracts for every work?

Institutional Performance Measures

With a focus on quantitative approaches, the construction of physical facilities has become an end in itself, losing sight of the primary objective—the delivery of water. Also noticeable are the involvement of local communities in their development and limited attention to operation and maintenance O&M issues. One of the main reasons for this is the dominant use of engineers and engineering expertise instead of multi-disciplinary inputs like finance, management, economics and sociology. Engineers dominate the PHEDs and boards. Their expertise is in the hardware components of water supply. For example, in the revised project document of Ghogha Project in Gujarat (CMSU, 2001), it was observed that the main competence of GWSSB is mainly in the construction and O&M of regional schemes, individual schemes, and implementation of hand pump programmes. Therefore, the 'Gujarat Water Supply and Sanitation Board (GWSSB) is not the ideal agency to manage and implement projects with a strong focus on community management. GWSSB can, however, continue as an implementing agency for hardware water supply components'. It is therefore, essential to bring in multidisciplinary inputs to the WATSAN-sector reform efforts through involvement of NGOs and private sector.

Transfer of Funds, Functions and Functionaries

The 73rd and 74th Amendments to the Indian Constitution included drinking water and sanitation in the list of 29 functions transferred to the local self-governments or PRIs. The state governments were supposed to transfer WATSAN functions to the local self-governments on the principle of 'functions, functionaries and funds should go together'. Even the Kerala government, which had tried to implement this principle, could not succeed in WATSAN sector. The PRIs were willing to accept the funds and functions, but not the high-cost functionaries of Kerala Water Authority. In any case, the engineers of the Kerala Water Authority were strongly against being transferred to PRIs. In most other states, neither the funds nor the functionaries in the WATSAN sector are being transferred to PRIs. What is being transferred are the schemes and pilot projects implemented as part of the WATSAN-sector reform efforts.

Inadequate Funding and Poor Pricing

Water is an economic resource. It is no longer a free resource. It is no longer abundant, and is going to get scarcer by the day. It costs money to develop it, process it, make it potable, distribute it, and manage it. The total capital requirement to cover all the rural habitations to supply of 40 lpcd of safe drinking water by restoring functionality or rehabilitating the existing systems would require Rs. 170–200 billion (World Bank, 1999). That is an allocation of Rs. 17–20 billion per year for the next 10 years. Only 3–5 per cent of these funds are expected to come from external sources. Possibilities of private investments are limited due to high risks, long payback period, and low profitability. The public contribution to capital cost of WATSAN services is yet to take root in India. Very little is done in the implementation of recovery of O&M costs, even though it is accepted as a policy.

Even where water charges are levied, they are nominal—never at a level to recover the capital costs. In Gujarat, some of the rural water supply schemes cover as long as 200 km. Electricity charges alone cost as much as Rs. 50–100 per person per year, but only Rs. 14 is charged. For even individual schemes, electricity charges are fully paid by the government. This is true, at present, even in the pilot project districts covered under RGNDWS. In addition, Rs. 15,000–30,000 is paid every year as O&M costs for each panchayat. Most village panchayats charge Rs. 100–150 per year per household, but not even 5 per cent is actually recovered (GSDWIC, 2000).

The recovery of costs is a complex issue. It has political, sociological, managerial, and operational complexities. Most PRIs do not have adequate staff with the capability to deal with these complexities. However, people will pay in case the village level arrangements for drinking water supply, meet their demands. It is interesting to note that in a village with a population of 2,000 in Ropar taluka in Gujarat, about 300 water pouches of 250 ml each at the rate of Re. 1.00 per pouch are sold every day during the summer months of May and June. If people can pay for pouch water, why not for regional water supply? It was found in the study that the people were willing to participate in the rural water and sanitation programmes by providing labour, monetary contribution, looking after maintenance and management of the system in the village. However, in most villages, people would require capacity building for carrying out these responsibilities.

The Missing Link Between Sanitation and Drinking Water

The pilot projects initiated by RGNDWS in 1997 and the recently launched Swajaldhara Programme are part of the WATSAN sector reforms. The responsibility for management and operation of rural sanitation, including waste disposal, environmental sanitation, and storm drainage are the responsibilities of the PRIs. These are funded under the employment generation programme and hence not properly integrated with the water supply programme. Recently, the responsibility for implementing sanitation programmes was transferred to rural development departments from the PHEDs and water supply departments. The separate institutions for sanitation (like sanitation authority/board) created at the state level further increases the distance between sanitation and drinking water programmes.

A Fragmented Approach

Not only are water supply and sanitation functions not properly integrated, but even the drinking water supply activities are not linked with water conservation and watershed programmes (Hordijk et al., 2002) as if they have no consequence for drinking water. It is well known that village tanks, ponds and lakes are not only sources of irrigation but also important sources of ground water recharge. Even the irrigation canals can be an important source of ground water recharge (Sakthinadivel and Chawla, 2003).

Rainwater harvesting is an important option to solve India's water problems. If India uses 3.65 million hectares of land or a little more than 1 per cent of its total land area for rainwater harvesting, it can get us 40 billion cubic metres of water per year, which is 4 per cent of the total estimated utilizable water resources. This is just to show the vast potential that rainwater harvesting holds for our country, which is fortunately endowed with good average rainfall. The significance of rainwater harvesting lies in the context of the critical situation of the groundwater resources. Taking the world scenario, only 1.6 per cent of all the liquid sweet water resources that exist at any point of time are to be found in rivers, lakes and swamps—the remaining 98.4 per cent of fresh water exists in the form of moisture and groundwater. In India, the use of groundwater has grown explosively since the 1950s. As a consequence, water tables are dropping. Saline intrusion has also become a problem in many coastal regions. Depletion of static groundwater reserves is a well-known problem in some areas such as Mehsana district in Gujarat, Coimbatore district in Tamil Nadu, and Kolar district in Karnataka (Pant, 2003).

There is a need to consider rainwater as a source. So far ground water and surface water are considered as sources. Roof-top rainwater harvesting is essential for all urban areas. This should be made mandatory and building by-laws should be amended accordingly. Chennai and Ahmedabad have taken a lead in this regard, and their example needs to be replicated in all cities.

This fragmented approach and multiplicity of organizations involved in the WATSAN sector activities is resulting in avoidable delays and unsatisfactory performance. For example, it took almost three years for the Gujarat government to decide who should implement RGNDWS pilot projects—the GWSSB, the rural development department or the Panchayati Raj department. Ultimately, the GWSSB is implementing the pilot projects.

Inadequate Attention to Sanitation

The Centrally Sponsored Rural Sanitation Programme (CRSP) was launched in 1986 with the objective of improving the quality of life of the rural people and to provide privacy and dignity to women. The concept of sanitation was expanded in 1993 to include personal hygiene, home sanitation, safe water, garbage and excreta disposal and waste water disposal. The components of the programme include construction of individual sanitary latrines for households below the poverty line (BPL), conversion of individual sanitary latrines, construction of village sanitary complexes for women, setting up of sanitary marts, intensive campaign for awareness creation and health education.

While demand for water has become a central issue, hygiene and sanitation are yet to acquire social and political priority (GSDWIC, 2000). Improvement in hygiene is impossible without a safe drinking water source and a safe means for disposal of excreta. This is going to happen not by issuing guidelines and government orders, but by bringing behavioural change at individual and community levels.

Sustained efforts and investments in information, education and communications (IEC) are essential to bring about this change. As mentioned earlier, government departments are poorly equipped to undertake this responsibility.

To overcome this problem, the Government of India and some state governments had restructured the Central Rural Sanitation Programme and launched it as Total Sanitation Campaign (TSC) that in 1999 as part of the Ninth Plan. The campaign was launched in project mode in 150 identified districts throughout the country (Chandra, 2001). But the government is still using the carrot of subsidy, which itself is reduced from Rs. 2,000 per unit to Rs. 500 per unit for BPL households. Though the government recognizes that the poor coverage of sanitation was due to emphasis on hardware and targets (Chandra, 2001), the subsidies and the financial outlay invariably lead to the target-oriented approach.

WATSAN REFORM EFFORTS IN GUJARAT

It is interesting to note that a number of community models are available in a number of states in the country. For instance, the Midnapore model of O&M of hand pumps has been recognized as a good model worth being adopted by other states. In this model, a water committee is established in the village and two women from the community are trained as caretakers. As for the monetary aspect, each beneficiary contributes Rs. 500 as initial fund for the hand pump and thereafter Re. 0.50 per month towards maintenance. This model is being observed as a wholly self-sustaining model. Local NGOs have also played an important role in the success of this model. Several such models exist, but most of them are addressing only a part of the problem—distribution of water, O&M of water structures and hand pumps, sanitation, and rainwater harvesting, etc. There is a need to integrate all the activities. The Water and Sanitation Organisation (WASMO) of Gujarat is such a model.

The creation of WASMO, as a registered society, is a major milestone. This was preceded by several important studies in the water sector—the white paper on water (IRMA, 2001), *Jal-Disha 2010* (GSDWIC, 2000) and the hydrological regimes study sponsored by the Gujarat Ecology Commission in 2000.

The WASMO Model .

The creation of WASMO is an important institutional development in the WATSAN sector (IRMA, 2002). The model recommends complete decentralization of WATSAN functions to the *pani samiti* or village panchayats. According to the model, the GWSSB would have responsibility for regional WATSAN schemes; it would bring water, wherever possible and necessary, to the boundary of the village. The WATSAN structures and functions within the village would be undertaken by the *pani samiti*. The state government would provide funds for the capital works, villagers contributing at least 10 per cent of the cost of such works. The entire O&M expenses would be borne by the *pani samiti*. Similarly, all the sanitation works in the village would be undertaken by the *pani samiti*. The main principles of the WASMO model are:

- Community-managed implementation of in-village water and sanitation improvements with village communities fully involved in and responsible for all stages of this process;
- Institutions facilitating support for the development of management capacity within communities receiving programme support.

It is believed that the application of these features will enable decentralization of the water and sanitation sector involving the transfer of 'ownership' and management to the village/panchayat community. Main components of the WASMO model are discussed in the following sections.

Water Supply Security

The programme addresses the full range of possible water sources for each village. This can involve pipe supply from a GWSSB regional scheme, a local panchayat-managed pipe supply, open village wells, village tanks and other lesser sources. This is to ensure that every village has access to secure water supplies and facilities. This involves continuity and security of supply with built-in drought proofing for villages from the integrated use of multiple sources (when available), and with choice and design of structures and facilities for earthquake resistance in earthquake-prone areas. For both, flexible planning and design are required. Provision of a minimum secure supply of drinking quality water will be supplemented with other sources of lesser quality for alternative uses.

Village Sanitation

The reportedly low level of sanitation and hygiene awareness and interest need to be enhanced for achieving greater community support for sanitation improvement. This could be achieved through a programme on hygiene awareness promotion and hygiene education for improved management of household water and waste management hygiene within the villages. The underlying requirement will be to stimulate better understanding of the significance of improved village hygiene with a fundamental shift in attitudes in favour of better sanitation and improved hygiene practices within communities. Primary objectives of sanitation and hygiene improvement activities will be to:

- Raise the awareness of village communities and households to existing sanitation problems and deficiencies;
- Promote the development of a 'community conscience' for cleaner more hygienic conditions in the communal areas of villages;
- Work to improve personal and household hygiene practices in relation to household water use and storage, household cleanliness and personal hygiene and defecation practices;
- Support the introduction of practical solutions and sanitation improvements and facilities for both the community and households; and
- Promote the conservation and recycling of personal wastes and reuse of household wastewater and wastes through gardening, composting and similar practices

Community Involvement

The WATSAN activities will target the whole village community involving all groups and both genders. With the existing limitations of village social structures, it is necessary that there should be truly democratic involvement of all villagers, without the exclusion of peripheral and/or marginalized groups. This means including the 'voices' and needs of the 'voiceless' while ensuring a room for their unequivocal participation during all stages of the in-village community management process. The needs and priorities of community women as the most vulnerable target group will be given special focus. This will include their active involvement in the organization and activities of village-level institutions like the *pani samitis*.

WASMO aims to build on the existing inherent capacity of community members to manage their private businesses (largely agricultural) and personal affairs. It will assist village communities with the development of a more structured panchayat-related organization—*pani samiti*. In exceptional cases where *pani samitis* cannot be formed for whatever reasons, WASMO could work with the village panchayat. WASMO will help the *pani samiti* to acquire additional expertise and capacity to enable them to develop, implement and manage their own integrated water and sanitation activities. For this, WASMO will need to gain the confidence of the *pani samiti* and establish a supportive 'partnership' based on mutual trust.

Programme Facilitating Support

The establishment of effective *pani samitis* in the villages will require facilitating support. Facilitation support to *pani samitis* will require the involvement of a large number of NGOs in the programme. Selected NGOs with proven capacity and credibility in the area will be assigned the task of providing support to the *pani samiti*. The NGOs will have no direct implementation responsibility, which will be vested in each *gram sabha*/village community. The Engineering Support Cell, comprising empanelled engineers (both retired and those not in service), will provide the technical support to the *pani samitis*. The WASMO head office will be responsible for overall coordination through development of programme facilitation guidelines, appropriate operational procedures and monitoring systems. WASMO will need to discharge its coordination responsibilities through its field units to be set up under the programme.

For effective support, it will be essential that a common overall approach and methodology is developed and applied by all the selected NGOs and a team-approach developed with the engineers and village organizations. In practice, however, variations in application detail will occur and will be accepted as an important part of the learning process – feedback of experiences and lessons.

Sector Policy and Development

The water and sanitation programme in each district will be implemented as only one of WASMO's wider sector responsibilities and activities. Hence, each district-level programme's innovative concepts of decentralized facilitated community managed development of community water and sanitation will be a valuable source of experience and provide lessons for the sector. WASMO will pool these innovative experiences, synthesize and feed to the policy initiatives of the government.

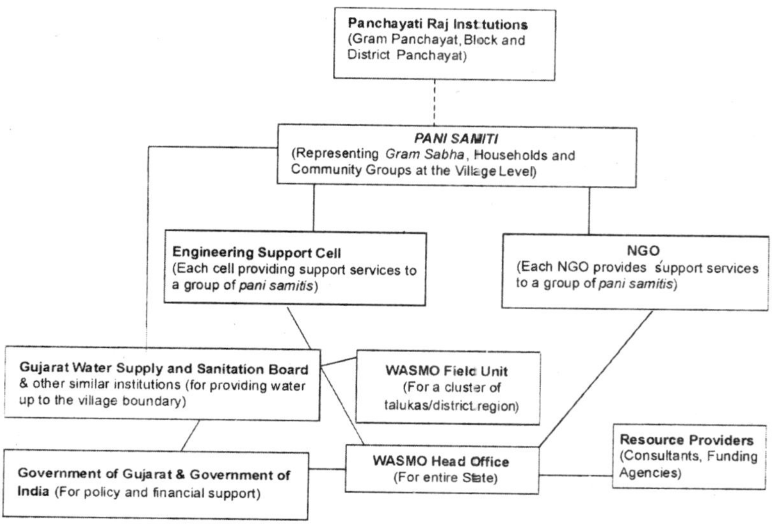

Fig. 5.2: Organogram of Water and Sanitation Management Organization.

The *pani samiti* is the core of the WASMO model of water and sanitation programme, together with the gram sabha and the households and community groups they represent. The village *pani samiti* will be a subcommittee of the village panchayat, but it will be a broader group drawing its members from each social group in the village, including women, SC/ST, minorities and other disadvantaged groups. Village-level or other local specialists and stakeholders could also be included in the *pani samiti*. Local-level political processes will also be a consideration in forming the *pani samitis*. The field workers of the supporting NGO will assist in capacity building of the *pani samiti* members. Additionally, *pani samitis* could draw support from the taluka and district panchayats, GWSSB and other resources providers.

The *pani samiti* will directly receive grants from WASMO. It will be accountable to the village panchayat, gram sabha and WASMO for the funds received and their proper utilization in accordance with the Village Action Plan. The Government of Gujarat will need to pass a resolution empowering the village *pani samitis* to directly receive grants from government, WASMO and others for undertaking water- and sanitation-related improvement activities. This will be in consequence to the earlier 1995 Government of Gujarat resolution (PRCH 1095-941/ch) providing for the formation of *pani samitis* to undertake water- and sanitation-related activities at village level. The roles of *pani samitis* will be built on those already provided for in the above government resolution. The significant roles of the *pani samitis* will be as follows:

- Ensure that issues of water supply, sanitation and water resources management are taken up with the gram sabha;
- Ensure that a Village Action Plan is prepared and approved by the WASMO field unit for all programme-supported activities;
- Ensure that the community is involved at all stages of planning, design, arranging, implementation, monitoring and management of water supply, sanitation and water resources management improvements;
- Organize and/or procure construction materials, labour and the services of engineers and contractors required for water supply, sanitation and water resources management improvement works;
- Organize, supervise and monitor construction and other programme activities;

- Ensure that the community makes contributions in cash, kind, materials and so on;
- Open a bank account to receive funds, in particular contributions from the community and others;
- Overall management of village programme finances;
- Keep accounts of programme and community money received and expenditures incurred;
- Report on the completion of all works and establish systems for the ongoing use and care of village water and sanitation systems;
- Spread awareness and consciousness about water usage and charges throughout the community;
- Consciously include women in day-to-day affairs and the use and care of systems and resources by encouraging them to become involved as members of the *pani samiti* and in other village activities involving the programme;
- Support the regular monitoring of activities by the NGO and the WASMO field unit.

The model is currently being implemented but not all policy principles are being adhered to as many of its staff are on deputation from government departments.

CONCLUSIONS

Unlike in other WATSAN reform efforts where only the demand management is being emphasized, the WASMO model suggests an integrated approach to the WATSAN programme, i.e. water conservation, water harvesting, and water supply and demand management. Many NGOs and even individuals are making similar interventions throughout India. While such efforts are extremely important, their coverage is limited and their sustainability in the absence of funding support to them is doubtful. Therefore, it is essential that local self-government institutions like village panchayats have to be empowered and their capacities increased to take up WATSAN functions. The WASMO model attempts to precisely do this and at a very large scale. The state government, with the support of Royal Netherlands Embassy, plans to implement the WATSAN sector reforms in the next 5–10 years throughout the state. The WASMO head office and its field units will provide the much needed coordination, information support, and programme implementation support to the *pani samitis*. If the WASMO field units function properly, they can become field laboratories, and providing valuable insights into WATSAN sector issues. Much will depend on whether in doing so the original design and principles will be adhered to.

REFERENCES

Hordijk, A., C van Wijk and K.P. Reddy, 'Report of Institutional Support Mission': Andhra Pradesh Academy of Rural Development (APARD), Utrecht: Matrix Consultants, 2002.

Ballabh, V., 'Governance in Water Resources, Issues, Challenges and Strategies', unpublished report, Anand: IRMA, 2003.

Chandra, Satish, 'A New Strategy for Sanitation: Linking Water and Health in the Central Rural Sanitation Programme', *Jalvani*, vol. 4, no. 1, 2001, p. 5.

CMSU, 'Ghogha Regional Water Supply and Sanitation Project', revised project document, Gandhinagar: Narmada Water Resources and Water Supply Department, Community Management Support Unit, 2001.

Government of India, Draft working group report on rural water supply and sanitation for the Formulation of Ninth Five Year Plan, New Delhi: Rajiv Gandhi National Drinking Water Mission, 1997.

———, 'Water Resources Development Plan of India: Policy and Issues', New Delhi: Ministry of Water Resources, 1999.

———, Ministry of Rural Development, Department of Drinking Water Supply: Accelerated Rural Water Supply Programme, New Delhi: Office of the Comptroller and Auditor General of India. http://cagofindia.delhi.nic.in/cag/reports/union/rep2002/2002_civil3/chapter3.pdf, 2002.

———, *India Economic Survey 2002-03*, New Delhi: Ministry of Finance, 2003.

GSDWIC, *Gujarat Jal-Disha 2010*, Ahmedabad: National Institute of Design, Gujarat State Drinking Water Infrastructure Company, 2000.

IRMA, White Paper on Water in Gujarat, Anand: Institute of Rural Management, 2001.

———, Mission and Organisation Structure for Water and Sanitation Management Organization (WASMO), Part 1, Anand: IRMA, 2002.

Pant, K.C., *India's Development Scenario: Next Decade and Beyond*, New Delhi: Academic Foundation, 2003.

Sakthinadiovel, R. and A.S. Chawla, 'Innovations in Conjunctive Water Management: Artificial Recharge in Madhya Ganga Canal Project', Baramulla: International Water Management Institute, 2003.

WHO/UNICEF, Joint Monitoring Programme for Water Supply and Sanitation Coverage Estimates 1980-2000, www.childinfo.org/oddb/water/asia/india_water, 2003.

World Bank, *Rural Water Supply and Sanitation: India Water Resources Management*, New Delhi: Allied Publications, 1999.

CHAPTER 6

People's Initiatives for Sustainable Solutions: Water Harvesting and Management in Gujarat

NAFISA BAROT

INTRODUCTION

Two diametrically opposite approaches are seen at work in the western Indian state of Gujarat for providing a sustainable solution to the ever increasing shortage of drinking water. One approach touts the multi-billion-rupee dam on the Narmada River as the panacea. It suggests the construction of canals and the laying of pipelines as the surest way to quench the thirst of a parched hinterland. The emphasis in this approach is on capital intensive technology, centralized planning and control, and commercialization of water to trigger off an agricultural and industrial revolution. The government plans to spend over Rs. 20,000 million, more than € 500 million, to supply drinking water to over 12,000 villages through a pipeline from the Narmada River. The other approach favours finding local solutions by the local people. The emphasis in this approach is on tapping rainwater where it falls, harvesting surface run-off, recharging groundwater resources, promoting conservation, economic use and equitable distribution, and enhancing management and control by the user communities.

Utthan, an independent non-government agency, is a protagonist of the people-centred approach. This paper sets out the urgency of community-based and people-centred policies and actions and presents the experience on which this commitment is based. Today there is a wider acceptance of this approach, not just among other NGOs that are active in tackling the issue of drinking water, but also in the policy documents of the state and central governments. At the international level, Vision 21 (WSSCC, 2000), the recommendations on freshwater in Bonn (GTZ, 2001) and the WEHAB sector approach that emerged in Johannesburg all call for genuine empowerment of local people to find local solutions in which equity is the key and access a human right. Yet the realities on the ground show how difficult it is to move from rhetoric to practice.

WATER CONDITIONS AND INTERVENTIONS IN GUJARAT

The peninsular region in Gujarat represents a classic case of how the indiscriminate use of groundwater for the cultivation of cash crops, the vagaries of nature in the form of cyclonic storms and droughts, and the rapid growth of industries have together turned a once fertile area into a highly saline and barren plane. The developments have led to the pauperization of the socially disadvantaged original inhabitants and have made them vulnerable to malnutrition and fluorosis. With landownership and control in the hands of rich landlords, poor men have been forced to migrate to the cities and to other states in search of employment. Meanwhile, the women have to fetch water from faraway places, often trekking four to five kilometres to and from the water source each day. They are further burdened by their tasks of collecting wood for fuel and fodder for cattle, two other natural resources that have become equally scarce as drinking water.

Interventions by the state government have not only failed to solve the problem, but have actually compounded it. Most interventions have benefitted the socially and politically powerful villages, leaving the remaining ones to fend for themselves. Government-sponsored schemes of supplying drinking water through pipelines and tankers are expensive and non-sustainable and have triggered off violent conflicts, bred corruption and increased gender inequalities. Due to a well-entrenched patriarchal and feudal system that governs the functioning of local government, the panchayats (elected local councils) have failed to give people access to the basic needs for their survival, such as water, fuel and fodder.

A group which is particularly badly affected are the Adivasis, who live in the Aravali range of hills spread across southern Rajastan, western Madhya Pradesh and north-eastern Gujarat. Once, these hills were covered by dense forests which provided the Adivasis with all their needs. However, from the start of the nineteenth century onward, the forests were cut down for the construction of houses and railways and for use in the furniture industry. Over the years the balded hills became scarred with mine pits from which the government and the private mining industries extracted limestone and other minerals. With market pressures increasing, the former forest dwellers were forced into seasonal 'distress' migration to the cities in search of work and food. The rich ecosystem which sustained them for centuries stands ravaged today.

The pressure on natural resources has heavy and negative impacts on women. Although female literacy has improved, it is still nowhere near the level of male literacy. Politically, women's opportunities have improved as well, with reservations for them in Panchayats. However, with lower educational levels and little exposure to the outside world, women are as yet not fully able to utilize these opportunities. The system of patriarchy is still strong and resisting the advancement of women. The worsening gender ratio in the state is an indicator of the growing preference for boys and brings with it a trend of rising violence against women, female foeticide and suicides. Women's productive roles in farming and animal husbandry, and their collection of household water and fuel wood go largely unrecognized in the state's economy.

INITIATING A PEOPLE'S MOVEMENT

Over twenty years ago, Utthan began its intervention in the saline and barren Bhal region in Ahmedabad district. Feudal practices had left women with little power to direct their own lives or to contribute effectively to community well-being. Violent conflicts over scarce drinking water were a daily affair and inhibited collective action. The government had an ambitious plan to supply drinking water to this region through a pipeline and tankers. The proposed schemes were unsustainable and would have led to the accentuation of conflicts between groups with vested interests and the underprivileged, as a group of powerful men dominated the socio-political institutions in the area. If water was brought to the area through pipelines and tankers, the same powerful group would have had absolute control over the resource.

Utthan started community organization among the women and the other underprivileged groups in the area. A vibrant women's movement emerged and led to the creation of a women's organization, Mahiti. The women formed village water committees which began to manage the communal water resources, first through the protection of ponds and then by augmentation of water availability through rainwater harvesting. In every committee at least one third of the members are women. The movement also compelled the government to support the development of local drinking water resources and ensured equity in the distribution of the water.

Armed with this experience, Utthan moved to the adjoining districts of Bhavnagar and Amreli. To start, opportunities were created for women and men to share their concerns and ideas, and gradually set their own agendas and realize their own potential. Most local problems were related to water scarcity. In due course, the communities in the two new districts started local rainwater harvesting systems and constructed check dams that could conserve precious rainwater and recharge wells and the aquifer. In each village, the location of the sites for the development of new water resources was selected in consultation with geologists and the village water committees. The groups also improved household and environmental sanitation and benefitted from new water- and agriculture-related employment opportunities.

Today, the movement has extended into Gujarat's urban areas, where the rapid pace of urbanization encounters critical conditions of scarcity, squalor and deprivation of every kind. A demonstration project on urban rainwater harvesting is now underway in the state capital of Ahmedabad, with the collaboration of a range of scientific, technical and administrative agencies.

Since the village water committees implement all activities related to water resources development, Utthan's role is only that of a facilitator and consultant. It organizes training workshops, exposure visits and awareness drives for members of water committees. In doing so, Utthan builds on the basic principles of Mahatma Gandhi of finding local solutions to basic livelihood through people's participation in decisions and resolution of conflicts through consensus. Utthan finds these principles as relevant, if no more, as they were nearly half a century ago.

RESULTS AND IMPACTS

Today, more than one hundred villages have put up alternative natural resources management systems and have shown that the followed approach can go to scale. The capacity building efforts have enabled women and other members of the water committees to understand technical, financial and logistic aspects of water resource management. Since the people of the villages involved take their own planning decisions, carry out their own construction and management and also make financial contributions to the projects, a strong feeling of ownership for the water resources has developed among them.

In 2000–1, a total of 20 watershed development projects involving a capital outlay of over Rs. 40 million (c. € 1 million) were completed under the National Watershed Development Programme. In addition to this, nine watershed projects were undertaken under the Integrated Wasteland Development Programme, involving a capital outlay of over Rs. 12 million. Utthan is further responsible for implementing another 23 watershed projects under the national programme in the districts of Dahod, Bhavnagar and Amreli. The National Bank for Agriculture and Rural Development (NABARD) co-finances the implementation of another five projects in Dahod district involving an outlay of over Rs. 10 million.

The monetary value of the participation of the villagers in the completed watershed developments amounts to Rs. 2.4 million for their labour alone, without calculating the value of their time for local planning and management. To the NABARD project, they have contributed voluntary labour worth over Rs. 90,000. In Rajula taluka, the villagers volunteered to repair check dams damaged during heavy monsoon rains.

In fluoride affected Balisana village in Patan district, women led a rainwater harvesting effort that can recharge and store up to 320 million litres of water per year, enough to provide the village with fluoride-free water for domestic use over the next two years. Community-mobilized resources covered 40 per cent of the total costs of Rs. 7.5 million. In addition, the community has put innovate arrangements in place to regulate the proper use of the water and has withstood considerable pressure from vested interest groups to gain control over the water for commercial use.

Calculations of the construction of locally planned, built and managed water supply systems show that their average cost amounts to Rs. 1,500 per inhabitant. The comparable cost of multi-village piped water supplies constructed by the government is Rs. 5,000 per capita.

So far, 75 per cent of the 108 villages in the four districts have become self-reliant for the supply of their drinking water because of the alternative systems of water resources developed by them. Earlier, women of these villages had to walk long distances to fetch drinking water, and during the scarcity period the government had to supply water imported through tankers from far off places.

The success which the women's movement has achieved is evidenced by the experiences in the drought of 2002. By using a comprehensive approach of check dams, farm ponds, well recharging percolation tanks, wastewater weirs, hand pump recharge and roof rainwater harvesting, sufficient water was stored to meet basic household needs for over two years.

There has also been a substantial increase in the income of families living below the poverty line as women are able to engage in farm and non-farm activities, now that they have been freed from the burden of fetching drinking water. Enhanced possibilities to produce fodder and fuel-wood around the homes free women further for other economic, domestic and community work. There has been a marked decline in the migration of people from both the coastal and tribal project villages as they were able to find gainful employment in their own or nearby villages following the introduction of an additional crop season.

The most visible impact of the comprehensive project approach has been on the health of women and children and the general cleanliness of the villages. None of the villages in the projects had any primary health care facilities. Visits by government health workers were also limited. Water scarcity affected personal hygiene and lowered food production and nutrition levels. Gender discrimination in health care and nutrition cut across caste and class differences as women's health needs had the lowest priority. Traditionally, for example, the women have to eat after the men and the children. As a result, many women suffer from anaemia and bear underweight children. Women are often the victims of wrong diagnosis, and reliance on local witchdoctors is not uncommon. Utthan initiated work in basic health care, hygiene and sanitation. It trained local health workers and linked them to the primary health centres. Awareness camps were organized in schools and community centres. With a view to popularizing local alternative systems of medicine such as ayurveda, homeopathy and yoga, farmers received training in growing medicinal plants and ayurveda practitioners met in workshops. Families now protect their drinking water from contamination and use a ladle to draw water from the pots. Children are washed, combed and their nails regularly cut. Villages where people formerly dumped garbage near water sources have now identified alternative sites for solid waste disposal. Households have made soak pits for waste water disposal outside the houses. This has made the streets cleaner and has reduced sites for insect breeding during the dry season. Inclusion of bathing places for women has also contributed to better hygiene and health conditions in a hot climate. Skin and eye infections have been reduced.

INFLUENCING POLICY

Utthan has been playing a key role in advocating the cause of people's participation in planning, execution and management of various development schemes in the state, with gender and social equity as central principles. A major step towards promoting the cause of participatory and decentralized water resources management systems has been the formation of Pravah, a state-level network of over 80 NGOs, technicians, scientists, research organizations and other institutions working on issues of drinking water and sanitation. Most of its member NGOs are involved in implementing various drinking water and sanitation schemes in the state and are in close contact with the concerned state and central agencies.

The state government consults Utthan from time to time in matters related to gender issues, e.g. women's empowerment, women's health and women's participation in water and other natural resources management. Utthan was instrumental in forming Mahila Swaraj Abhiyan (MSA), a state-level network of NGOs working on women's issues. MSA held a state-level conference of elected women members of local government institutions to share experiences and discuss the challenges that women members of local bodies for self-government face. Utthan is further a member of a network of women's organizations in the Saurashtra and Kutch regions formed to launch a campaign against violence on women. The network has carried out an education drive among rural women to make them aware of their rights and of laws to prevent such violence. At the national level, Utthan is a member of Rashtriya Jal Bidari, a forum of voluntary organizations and individuals that advocates decentralized water resources management; of Catch Water, a national movement initiated by the Centre for Science and Environment (CSE) in New Delhi; and of the National Water Harvesters Network. The Executive Trustee of Utthan is a nominated member of the Expert Group on Political Participation and Empowerment of Women which the Government of Gujarat set up in 2002. She represented the NGO sector at the All India Conference on the Role of the Voluntary Sector in National Development inaugurated by Prime Minister Atal Behari Vajpayee on 20 April 2002. Her keynote address received national attention and received specific reference in the prime minister's central message.

There have been strong examples from India and the South Asian subcontinent of achieving the goal of access to safe water for all. Yet there is great difficulty in going to scale with change because the policy makers and institutions in the water sector do not seem capable of taking up a real paradigm shift. Sustainability as a concept must respect the need for empowerment of and ownership by those most in need and progress should be judged by whether a real transfer of power is actually taking place.

The first major move towards a greater decentralization of water resources management in India took place through the work of the National Drinking Water Mission in the mid-1980s. The focus of the gigantic effort to bring safe water to millions of citizens was the hand pump. Despite major achievements, the goals of adequate access and coverage still remain unmet because of the ongoing depletion of water resources, the unresolved issues of the ownership of these resources and the inadequacy of meeting the goals through any single technology such as the hand pump.

More recently, India initiated a Sector Reform Programme, in which the emphasis was once more on decentralized water supplies, implemented and managed by local institutions, in particular village water committees and gram panchayats. The Swajaldhara programme, which is the latest extension of sector reforms, stresses direct access to central resources by local institutions. Simultaneously, rainwater harvesting is assuming a greater importance as water tables fall further and survival in many parts of the country depends on the ability to catch water where it falls.

Utthan's experience in Gujarat has been twofold, cooperating with state agencies to implement these central government initiatives and undertaking independent projects through civic society. Its work at state level has focussed on establishing viable water and sanitation committees in villages, tracking the progress of massive pipeline schemes linked to the Narmada River project and participation in a pilot project in Ghogha block of Bhavnagar district. In the latter, an experiment is underway to establish a model partnership between government systems, a donor and people's institutions. The project aims to cover a population of about 2,15,000 people in 82 villages. A recent development has been the setting up of a special institution, the Water and Sanitation Management Organization (WASMO), with assistance from the Netherlands, to oversee such partnerships in another five districts.

A significant reflection of growing partnerships has been the work of 30 NGOs and government institutions working together to develop a vision and action plan for Gujarat parallel to the Vision 21 report of the Water Supply and Sanitation Collaborative Council. Beginning at the same time as the WSSCC effort, the group formulated the *Jal-Disha 2010* report which included advocacy for policy change and which has received official as well as global acknowledgement.

While the progress is not inconsiderable, challenges and barriers to more rapid change continue. One problem is that in India, water and sanitation are state subjects. The central government can recommend and encourage but not enforce its national water policy. The latest policy furthermore raises concerns regarding interpretation and other policies. For example, it states that water is national property, while the then Prime Minister Atal Behari Vajpayee stated that water is the community's property. Implementation of sector reforms has been initiated in 65 districts across all states. In Maharashtra, Tamil Nadu, Karnataka, Uttar Pradesh and Andhra Pradesh, there is evidence of a clear political will to promote the initiative. In Gujarat, the experience has been disappointing. Communities have no genuine say in decision making. Instead of building local ownership over local resources and responding to local needs and capacities, the tendency is to recruit communities into serving central programmes imposed from above.

Institutional reform, so essential to change, is not taken seriously. Attitudes and systems geared to past mentalities are now expected to encourage decentralization and empowerment processes to which the institutions are not genuinely committed. An example is the decision to appoint elected village leaders, who hold a political position, to also head water and sanitation committees, rather than allowing users to choose their own water and sanitation leaders. In Ghogha, the state government insists on supplying Narmada water through pipelines up to the villages and to limit community participation to the distribution and management within the village boundaries. The communities, and especially the women, however, demand financial resources and support for planning their own local water supplies based on local potential.

The originally intended approach of autonomous state-level bodies to facilitate community participation and promote community-centred water and sanitation has now been abandoned. The new organizational structure, WASMO, is marked by bureaucratic control. At village level, NGOs have been advocating that women should represent at least half of its membership, that marginalized groups should be adequately included and that the communities should identify those willing and able to take up responsibilities for water and sanitation. Instead, the state has passed a resolution for the mandatory inclusion of politically elected officials, with the political head of the village, in charge. This does not allow the evolution of mechanisms for and culture of better governance. The Swajaldhara scheme that was launched in December 2002 leaves glaring questions about the space and scope for women's participation, for key institutional reforms, and for investment in capacity building at the grassroots.

CONCLUSION AND RECOMMENDATIONS

From a field perspective, the lack of genuine change is particularly frustrating because the need for genuine decentralization and local ownership as well as the strategy for how to achieve it has been spelled out in the *Jal-Disha 2010* report and was strongly ratified by experiences both in India and all over the world. The consensus on decentralization that emerged in The Hague and was subsequently endorsed in Bonn and Johannesburg is still far from being translated into a reality on the ground. Several steps are needed if the rhetoric is to become a reality:

- *Encourage local communities to undertake local solutions*: The achievements of a genuine paradigm shift have been clearly demonstrated over three years of drought in several districts in Gujarat.
- *Give priority to hygiene awareness and sanitation*: The overwhelming needs for better sanitation, hygiene and health can never be achieved unless linked to better water conservation, development and management and to the development of a local, gender-sensitive and women-led movement. As 50 years of experience indicates, hygiene cannot be imposed from the top. And without good hygiene and sanitation practices no amount of so-called safe water remains safe.
- *The urban crisis needs new capacities and approaches*: Experiences during the years since the Second World Water Forum in The Hague underline the need for those with predominant experience in rural development to pay increasing attention to the urban challenge by developing new approaches and by building the required capacity.
- *Paradigm shifts start in the minds and attitudes of the political and administrative leadership*: There is no way that established institutions working through their established systems can achieve the required change. New policies and new ways of doing things must be practised. Dramatic evidence of the dichotomy in Gujarat is that state policies and programmes continue to be based on the gigantic Narmada pipeline programme which is wholly government owned and operated. The only apparent space for local ownership is the distribution and management of water received from the central system without guarantee for or influence on actual delivery. The real need is for the bureaucracy to hand more power to local communities and this is proving a very difficult transfer. So long as the preoccupation with massive capital-intensive schemes continues,

there can be no genuine decentralization and local ownership. Most resources will be swallowed by the pipeline schemes and only marginal resources will be left to implement the people-centred approaches advocated at the global level in Vision 21 and in Gujarat by Pravah and the *Jal-Disha 2010* coalition.

- *Recognition and application of people's ownership of local water resources:* For stakeholders in India, the major need now is for national policies that clearly establish the ownership of local people over water resources that they can manage effectively. The state and local authorities then need to more uniformly apply this ownership, remove uncertainties which now surround issues of ownership and genuinely encourage people-centred projects on the ground. In 2003 a senior state official declared that every drop of rain falling from the sky belongs to the state. At the same time, those rich enough to dig deeper merrily exploit underground water resources. Genuine ownership of local resources will also require extremely close monitoring systems that can help ensure that key decisions are those of all users, and not of dominating power structures. Clear directives are also needed that ensure that financial resources are channelled to local community-led water resources development and management. A long-term programmatic commitment to improve and manage local water resources must be given by local, national and international governments and the communities themselves.
- *Acknowledge and support women's roles:* In all of the above, the state must acknowledge and support the roles of women in decision making, not just in rhetoric but through investment in capacity building and by building institutions in which women and other marginalized groups have the leading voice. Women should minimally represent half of the participants in all decision making and management processes at all levels.
- *Global responsibility to implement Vision 21:* Global stakeholders have a responsibility to ensure implementation of the principles of Vision 21 as well as the Bonn recommendations. The recent deliberations in Kyoto revealed that communities and authorities have made progress towards attaining these goals, but have also shown up the inadequacies of the achievements. There is clearly

no hope of achieving the Millennium Development Goals for safe water and sanitation if progress continues with the current pace and approaches. Policy and institutional reforms need to be jointly monitored by all partners. Donors may now need to examine ways in which their support can be accessed by those whose actions on the ground are in keeping with the principles of Vision 21 and thereafter. This may require major changes in policy to adequately reflect that governments must now be facilitators, not suppliers, and that other partners in civil society must be acknowledged as equals in the decision-making and implementation processes.

The focus on future partnerships must reflect a genuine shift towards local ownership for sustainability, the only paradigm that can work.

REFERENCES

WSSCC, Vision 21: Water for People: a shared vision for hygiene, sanitation and water supply and a framework for action, also forming the water for people component of the World Water Vision, Geneva: Water Supply and Sanitation Collaborative Council, 2000, http://www.wsscc.org/load.cfm?edit_id=45

GTZ, Republik of Germany, Federal Ministry for Economic Cooperation and Development and Federal Ministry for the Environment, Nature Conservation and Nuclear Safety, 'Water—A Key to Sustainable Development', Report of the International Conference on Freshwater, 2001, http://www.water-2001.de

WEHAB Working Group, 'A Framework for Action on Water and Sanitation', New York: United Nations Department of Economic and Social Affairs, Division for Sustainable Development, 2002, http://www.johannesburgsummit.org/html/documents/summit_docs/wehab_papers/wehab_water_sanitation.pdf

CHAPTER 7

Local Self-Government: Experiences in Madhya Pradesh and Challenges Ahead

YOGESH KUMAR

INTRODUCTION

Water has remained an important political issue as its availability or scarcity has a significant reflection on the quality of governance at national, state and local levels. The arguments of efficiency always favoured centralization in the delivery of water-related systems whereas those who believed in people's control over water argued for decentralization for long-term effectiveness and sustenance. In India, the enactment of the 73rd and 74th Amendments created a constitutional compulsion to devolve water management to the local bodies (GoI, 2004). The experiences with decentralization in the last ten years have been mixed as the already existing centralized systems of decision-making and delivery of programmes show little willingness to give away power and change their ways of operations (Johnson, 2003). On the other hand, many of the local self-governance bodies have demonstrated that community-based management of water can result in an effective utilization of the available external and internal resources (Kumar, 1996; Narain, 2003).

The last three decades in India are characterized by the enhancement of access to drinking water in remote areas and delegating its management to the communities as primary stakeholders. Appropriate technological options have emerged, such as the introduction of the India Mark-II/III hand pumps and micro piped water supply schemes and the renovation of traditional wells into safe drinking water sources. The 1980s and 1990s focused on building models of community managed water supply systems and sanitation. Examples of local water management committees are the Pani Panchayats in Rajasthan and the Jal Samitis in Uttar Pradesh (Kumar, 1996). Similar kinds of water user and management groups have been promoted in several other parts of the country. In some states, an office order of the concerned departments or the cabinet of ministers have recognized the value of these committees. However, such orders have a more limited impact for implementation than a constitutional mandate.

The experiments in many parts of India have demonstrated that people have the capacity to manage local water supply and sanitation issues by themselves. They have also provided the opportunity to explore and try out possible structures that fit into the existing top-down systems of water management. Efforts have been made to involve future and actual users and communities in the following activities:

- Selecting the sites for locating water points;
- Choosing appropriate designs for sanitary toilets;
- Carrying out preventive and curative maintenance of hand pumps; and
- Sharing responsibilities and authority to operate and maintain piped water supply systems.

The experiments have met with a number of challenges. A major challenge is rooted in the scarcity of resources along with the pressing need to reach large numbers of people with basic services. Issues of replication of successful experiments, therefore, become pertinent. Cost sharing and community-based management and maintenance have been undertaken especially to address the constraints in resources and realize ambitious coverage targets. In such situations, the *core* purpose of empowering communities often takes a backseat. In his paper on developing tools for assessing people's empowerment, Salil Shetty has stated that a large number of big projects have recommended community participation with the objective to recover cost and that very few projects have community empowerment as an objective.

This paper draws primarily on the experiences of community-managed water supplies and sanitation in Madhya Pradesh. This is one of the progressive states in India, which is working towards decentralization, experimenting with models of direct democracy and strengthening local self-governance institutions in rural and urban areas (Behar and Kumar, 2002). The paper also analyses the experiences in Madhya Pradesh with the Sector Reform Project, which is a pilot project of the Government of India to test out possible ways of transferring the control over water resources into the hands of local institutions including the Panchayati Raj Institutions, or PRIs (RGNDWM, 1999, 2002).

The non-governmental organization (NGO) Samarthan works in the district of Sehore to strengthen institutions of local self-governance. Its work is part of the Joint Action Programme initiated by Participatory Research in Asia (PRIA) for strengthening institutions of local self-governance. The initiative has so far spread to some 60 blocks in 13 Indian states. As water and sanitation are two of the primary needs for most communities, a water and sanitation programme was also launched. In Madhya Pradesh, SIDA and UNICEF support this initiative. The primary purpose of Samarthan has been to provide evidence of local institutional capacities in managing water and sanitation. This paper contains an analysis of the experiences in Sehore district where Samarthan has worked on the issues of water and sanitation along with urban and rural local self-governance institutions.

CONSTITUTIONAL AMENDMENTS FOR COMMUNITY MANAGEMENT OF WATER AND SANITATION

A decade ago, the Government of India adopted the 73rd and 74th Amendments to the Indian Constitution. The amendments recognized the legitimate role of the local government bodies elected by the citizens and their representatives at the village, town, city, block and district levels in enhancing economic development and social justice for their constituencies. The constitutional amendments have had serious implications for the management of development. The powers of decision-making as well as part of the resources for development, which so far had largely been controlled by the district administration, were devolved to the local bodies in the lower levels. The salient features of the 73rd Constitutional Amendment may be summarized as follows:

- Gram sabhas (general meetings of all voters) are held in each Panchayat as defined by law. A gram sabha meeting may be held with the voters of multiple villages within the panchayat or in each single village, depending on, e.g. the size of the population;
- A three-tier structure with district, block and community (gram) panchayat has been accepted. The members of these panchayats at all the levels are directly elected and not chosen by nominations;
- In all three tiers, seats are reserved proportionally to the size of the population at each level. More importantly, one-third of the total seats has been reserved for women;
- The Act ensures a five-year term for the PRIs. In the event of super session, new elections should be completed within six months from the date of dissolution;
- The state legislature has been given power to authorize panchayats to levy, collect and appropriate suitable local taxes and provide for making grants-in-aid to the panchayats from the consolidated fund of the state.
- In each state, a State Finance Commission will be set up once every five years to review and provide advice on the distribution of funds between the state and the local bodies;
- The state governments are to make legislations conforming the new amendments within a year from their adoption at the Central level;
- The Act devolved 29 development functions to panchayats, one of them being water and sanitation. It further indicated a set of items in the Eleventh Schedule of the Constitution, which the state government may entrust to the panchayats in addition to any other scheme for economic development and social justice. It has been envisaged that the transfer of funds, functionaries and functions to local bodies will strengthen panchayats at village and higher level and also help them provide efficient responses to local needs and enhance accountability to the voters.

The 73rd Amendment is considered a historical change. The Constitution now recognizes institutions for local self-governance, defines their autonomous roles and deepens the decentralization process (GoI, 2004). Various incentives have been given to the states for strengthening the PRIs. Some of the national funds are now directly devolved to the PRIs, so that they may exercise their power and implement development plans.

At the state level, the degree of recognition for and promotion of PRIs differs. Some states such as Madhya Pradesh, Karnataka and Kerala moved ahead whereas many others lagged behind. There is a strong relationship between the commitment of the state-level leadership to the constitutional reform and the degree of devolution of funds, functions and functionaries to the panchayats. The more supportive states have issued office orders and simplified guidelines to create more enabling environments for the PRIs.

The current panchayati raj system has now been in existence for 10 years and has provided an opportunity for the emergence of new leadership (Knight et al. 2002). Of the total number of panchayat representatives that have taken responsibilities, at least one-third are women. When sufficient support has been provided, many of them have performed their roles effectively The resources which have reached the village panchayats have been used more transparently and with a greater involvement of the village electorates, i.e. the gram sabhas (village assemblies). The latter has significantly enhanced the accountability of local institutions to the people.

Although the constitutional amendments provided the necessary conditions for a greater power of the panchayat institution, they did not, however, set down the operational details needed to provide a meaningful space for the panchayats to operate in (VANI, 1995). Examples of successful empowerment are limited and few, as the administrative machinery, policies and procedures are not quite conducive for panchayats to take charge of their own development. Moreover, the existing power equations, the skewed distribution of economic resources and the social hierarchy within the communities themselves have created serious impediments for panchayats to flourish and become self-reliant.

DEVOLUTION OF POWER TO GRAM SABHAS IN MADHYA PRADESH UNDER GRAM SWARAJ

Madhya Pradesh is one of the states in India, which headed the process of enacting the 73rd Amendment and organizing panchayat elections.

There have been two elections, each round for a term of five years. In 2000, Madhya Pradesh adopted a new Act for Gram Swaraj, which gave greater recognition to the villages as units of self-governance. The salient features of Gram Swaraj are the following:

- Each revenue village will be treated as an independent gram sabha instead of combining two or three villages in a larger entity as a village panchayat. The latter consists of a population of at least 5,000 people and combines a couple of villages;
- Each village will elect a treasurer who will be the village-level head for operating the village account within the panchayat;
- The gram sabha will constitute seven committees of eight to twelve members for health, education, infrastructure, agriculture, social justice, social security and public resources. The heads of these seven committees will constitute the Village Development Committee (VDC) with the Sarpanch as its head;
- Each committee will be responsible for planning and execution of development programmes in their respective sectors;
- The Health Committee can open an account for a water and sanitation programme and will be able to execute programmes related to health, water and sanitation;
- Each village within a panchayat will have its own account to which development resources provided to the whole panchayat will be transferred on a predetermined ratio;
- For reasons of social justice, half of the committee members will be from socially weaker sections and one-third of the seats will be reserved for women members.

IMPLICATIONS OF THE DEVOLUTION OF POWER

The proposed change in Madhya Pradesh has further decentralized power as citizens in small villages can now elect their own committees and make them more accountable than is possible in the much larger Panchayats. The model of the Gram Swaraj is an experiment to take the decentralization process beyond the democratic governance envisaged in the 73rd Amendment and bringing the centres of power closer to the people. For women, participation in smaller units of governance, especially in their own village, is both more feasible and effective as women find it difficult to travel even to the next village for participating in meetings. Their workload at home and lack of male support do not allow them to take part in meetings, which would require extra efforts and resources. Having the village as unit of governance is conducive to a greater participation and share in decision making by women and poor villagers.

However, in reality, social realities in villages are not developed enough and the citizens are not sufficiently aware to demand their rights and meaningfully discharge their responsibilities as peoples' representatives. The State Election Commission did not conduct the election of the committees under Gram Swaraj. Instead, either the village assemblies formed committees without sufficient understanding of the provisions, or they were the result of the joint decision of the Sarpanch and concerned government functionaries. Many of the citizens did not know that they had been nominated as members of various committees.

In many villages, the rule of a one-third proportion of women and socially deprived sections has not been maintained either due to ignorance or deliberately. Cross-checking of the lists of members is a difficult task as the new State Act may lead to over 4,50,000 committees. It would also require additional supervision and care to ensure that provisions related to social justice are practiced in letter and spirit.

The low levels of literacy and low awareness about the Act have also created constraints in the effective functioning of the committees. There is a need for building the capacities of the citizens and their committees on the operational aspects and develop their skills in planning and financial management.

The multiplicity of committees at the village level has furthermore made their respective charters unclear for the committee members. Water can be treated as a function under the health committee and the committees for infrastructure and public resources. The department has directed that water is a subject matter of the village health committee, but in many cases, conflicts of interests may not get resolved at the village level.

In spite of these difficulties, in many villages young treasurers have emerged as leaders and have challenged feudal leadership. Moreover, devolution of financial resources directly to panchayats has also given an opportunity to the villages for demonstrating their abilities to take control over their own problems, finding out solutions and implementing decisions. These experiences reflect the findings in the study of van Wijk and Garcia (2002) that better performing water supply systems were those where users were more informed and participated in project planning in a democratic manner, rather than schemes where users only shared the capital costs.

GRASSROOTS DYNAMICS

The 74th Amendment has also provided water management function to the urban local bodies. The Department of Water Works/Public Health Engineering has been transferred to urban local bodies. The bodies receive funds partially from the state government and partially from the collected water tax. Section 243-X of the 74th Amendment authorizes an urban local body to levy, collect and appropriate local taxes, duties, tolls and fees as per procedures. Similarly, the Twelfth Schedule of Article 243-W clearly lists water supply, public health, sanitation and solid waste management as areas under the jurisdiction of municipal bodies.

This shift in approach and devolution of power to the local bodies has generated a new dynamism at the community level among the development administration as well as the political leadership at the district and state levels (Kumar et al., 2001). The devolution of power and resources has a considerable impact on the water sector as it has enormous resources and much scope for maneuverability. Moreover, as water is a political issue, all influential political leaders and sitting MLAs and MPs want to take credit for providing water in their constituency. The many different stakeholders and the conflict of interest between them have made water one of the most contentious development issues.

One of the main programmes of the Government of India, the Sector Reform Programme (now called Swajaldhara), clearly contains the possibility that financial resources for drinking water and sanitation will directly flow to the gram sabhas and panchayats. Communities themselves must contribute about 10 per cent of the capital costs as a necessary condition to undertake water-related development work (RGNDWM, 2001). The status on the ground clearly reflects that the operational guidelines are not well specified. The willingness of the government machinery to give away responsibilities to the local bodies for planning, monitoring and implementation of their own water supply schemes is inadequate and the programme has therefore moved at a slow pace. Less than one-third of the allocated resources have been utilized in most of the districts of MP in the first two years of the programme. Methods to build community capacities to monitor their projects exist (PRIA, 2002), but are slow to be used in these programmes.

In the water sector, the recognition of panchayats and urban local bodies as legitimate institutions which make their own decisions and execute their own plans has obviously shaken up well-established administrative institutions that were overloaded with the management of water development projects and held absolute power in decision making, control and implementation of the water programme. Now, the Sector Reform Programme of the Government of India clearly recognizes the role of the gram sabhas and their committees in determining all needs related to water and sanitation. Local urban and rural bodies can make plans and implement water and sanitation schemes. A portion of the required investment funds can go directly to the village account along with guidelines for its expenditure. The role of the PHED and other departments is to facilitate and provide technical guidance. This shift in approach and strategies has visualized empowerment of urban and local bodies so that local institutions can implement water and sanitation schemes on a large scale and with efficiency and effectiveness. The effort of involving communities in planning and implementation will also lead to their active involvement in maintenance of the created water systems.

The creation of an enabling environment by enacting a positive policy framework has given the civil society organizations and other interested and well-meaning officials within the government a new handle to promote local institutions to perform their roles and responsibilities. However, the structural rigidities that exist within the system in the form of structures and functions of the departments, mechanisms of fund transfer and monitoring, and measures of performance assessment of the functionaries of the government are yet to be challenged and adapted to meet the growing demand for village water and sanitation projects that has emerged from the decentralization process.

COMMUNITY WATER MANAGEMENT: EXAMPLES

There are certain areas where urban and rural local self-governance bodies have moved ahead. In a number of communities, people have planned with collective wisdom and found appropriate solutions for their local context. A favourable policy environment has provided opportunities to panchayats and citizens to demand their rights.

The cases discussed in the following section give insight into the opportunities and bottlenecks which local bodies face with regard to water management. The purpose of highlighting such cases is primarily to identify areas that demand attention, such as improvements in institutional mechanisms, simplification of procedures and creation of a facilitative environment. Nevertheless, these examples also demonstrate the strengths of the communities and their institutions in managing their own affairs.

Case 1: Gram Sabha Evolves an Operation and Maintenance System

Thunakalan Panchayat consists of 500 families and is administratively divided into 16 wards. Four wards are outside the main settlement area. The panchayat had one tube well provided under a previous scheme, for which the panchayat had to pay the costs of maintenance and repairs. If this tube well was not working, many women and children had to go to the tube wells surrounding the village, the nearest at 2 km from the main habitation. This was a daily nuisance as the time involved could vary, severely affecting the everyday routine of the women for preparing food, getting the children ready for school and working in the field.

In April 2002, the panchayat received a bill of Rs. 5,000 for tube well operation, but it expressed itself unable to pay due to a paucity of resources. The sarpanch of the panchayat was an influential person and he managed to get the payment made by requesting the sitting MLA of the area to shell out the required amount from the MLA Local Area Development Fund. However, the MLA warned that this would be the last payment from his side.

Shanta Bai, a member of the local Self Help Group, raised the matter of the unsustained tube well within her group. She and her husband Pannalal were daily wage labourers working in the fields of the neighbouring villages. The husband–wife duo had to leave home everyday around eight, having first prepared their food for the day for themselves and their three children. Led by Shanta Bai, the women members of the SHG discussed the situation and decided that the maintenance system for the tube well had to be streamlined to the minutest detail. With this consensus, the women met the Panch of the ward, the treasurer of the gram sabha and finally a meeting was sought with the Sarpanch of the panchayat, Achal Singh Mewada. It was finally decided that the gram sabha meeting should be called with the issue being the prime agenda.

The gram sabha meeting was organized. In total, 213 members participated, exceeding the quorum requirement of 190, and 65 women took an active part. Estimates for the operation and maintenance cost of the tube well were worked out. It was decided that each of the benefitting families would pay Rs. 10 per month. Fifteen families opted for private connections with a monthly payment of Rs. 30. Each elected ward member was given the responsibility to collect the water charges from the families in his/her ward and to give them a receipt from a receipt book printed by the gram panchayat. They now collect the water tariff together with the payment for the electricity bill. Maintenance of the tube well takes place on a regular basis. The community has efficiently maintained the water supply for more than a year. The money collected is sufficient for regular maintenance of the tube well, periodic repairs and the payment of electricity bill. The managing committee has also decided that the tube well will be switched on for only two hours in the morning and in the evening. A tailoring shop next to the panchayat office is given responsibility to monitor the operation of the pump at the fixed times.

The woes of Shanta Bai and women like her were solved in this manner and the voice of the women folk of the village echoes in the words of the Anganwadi worker (nursery school teacher) of the village, Radha Bai. 'I need to arrange the Anganwadi centre very early in the morning. When the electricity connection to the tube well was cut, I myself had to go to the surrounding tube wells in the fields to fetch water. This became a hindrance to the successful running of the centre, in which many women used to leave their children during the time that they went to fetch water for their households. Now that the tube well has started functioning, the children are coming in larger numbers and at the scheduled time for their orientation towards schooling.'

Working upon the system further, the village has now developed an extension scheme for providing water supply to the outlying wards. The scheme has been submitted to the PHED for resources under the Sector Reform Programme. In another part of the state, there are similar examples of communities having developed their own systems of water management.

Case 2: A Community Plans and Implements its School Toilet Complex

In the village of Manpura where about 100 families live, there is a local government school with classes up to standard VIII. The school also caters to the demand of children from the neighbouring villages of Rola, Jakhakhedi and Rajukhedi, and the enrollment of girls is quite high. Nevertheless, the teachers felt that due to lack of toilets, their attendance and motivation were quite low. Particularly the girls who came from the neighbouring villages felt the lack of improper sanitation facilities. As one can expect, this came to the ears of the mothers and subsequently the issue of constructing a school toilet complex was raised in the gram sabha meeting. There was a consensus that a sanitation complex was needed, however, no action was undertaken due to a shortage of financial resources. Matters became worse when the treasurer of the local Self Help Group, Pushpa Bai, announced her decision to withdraw her elder daughter from the school because of her discomfort due to lack of proper school toilets.

The Child Environment Project in Madhya Pradesh, supported by the Swedish International Development Agency (SIDA) and UNICEF, had provisions for the construction of school toilets. Samarthan organized a village meeting and facilitated discussions on the felt need for a toilet by the community. There was an agreement to construct a toilet complex in the school with active participation of the community in its planning, implementation and monitoring.

A Water and Sanitation Committee was formed under the Gram Swaraj provisions. Matters took a positive turn when the gram sabha decided that women should constitute at least one-fourth of the total membership of the committee. A decision to this effect was immediately taken and four women were chosen as members of the twelve-person committee. The committee prepared a detailed plan, looked at the design aspects and worked out the costs. The plan was presented to the gram sabha and was approved and the decision recorded in the minutes. The responsibility of construction and purchase was clearly defined. The schoolteacher, assisted by the Anganwadi worker, Shyama Bai, was chosen to keep accounts on behalf of the committee.

This was the first time that the villagers were in the decision-making role during the planning and implementation of a development project. The processes and resources were transparent and known to everybody though the formal processes of the gram sabha. Every month, the committee presented its accounts in the assembly and informed the participants about the progress. This sustained the interest of the families so that they supported the committee in times of crisis. Another important aspect was the part played by the women members of the committee. Suhasini Chourasia, the president of the SHG in the village, who for a long time was the voice behind the women demanding the construction of the sanitation complex, took the lead in ensuring that the concerns of the fairer sex on the design of the toilet seats and their distance from the floor were met during the design of the complex. Savitri Bai, who lived close to the school, took charge of monitoring the quality of construction. Pushpa Bai, whose two daughters were enrolled in the school made her presence felt in the committee by bringing up the issue of the maintenance of the toilet. This led in later meetings to the resolution that for maintaining the cleanliness of the toilet, an additional Rs. 5 is to be charged per student per year as a contribution to the maintenance fund of the school. A sweeper will clean the toilet two days a week, charging Rs. 50 per week.

The small success of building the school toilet has increased the people's confidence to plan and implement their own development plans. Recently, the community has collected Rs. 25,000 and submitted a proposal for a piped water supply scheme costing Rs. 3,00,000 under the Sector Reform Programme. The experience of Manpura clearly reflects that the effective involvement of the community, and in particular the relevant stakeholders—in this case the mothers of the schoolgoing girl children—in planning and implementation builds up capacities to take up large initiatives for local development. The involvement of the panchayat and gram sabha made the processes transparent and accountable and were essential for long-term sustenance of the efforts as well as making it a democratic process.

Case 3: Procedural Delays in Accessing Resources under the Sector Reforms

In Bijora, just 7 km from Sehore town, Samarthan helped form two savings and credit groups two years ago. One of the groups consisted of Scheduled Caste members only, coming primarily from a Scheduled Caste-dominated hamlet. The village section with the dominant caste group had a hand pump where Scheduled Caste families were not allowed to draw water due to the local practice of discriminating untouchables. Women such as Rambha Bai, who was bedridden with a chronic disease, suffered the most. Her two children, one of whom was a student at the government school in the village and the other a daily wage labourer, had to spend their time fetching water for their house. During the summer, the single hand pump in the village was used day and night and families of Scheduled Castes were discriminated aganist, as they had to fetch water last after all the others.

When they heard about the Sector Reform Programme in the district, the SHG decided that their hamlet should have a separate hand pump. The women members decided to put the issue in front of the gram sabha at its next scheduled meeting. This time, the gram sabha of Bijora wore a different face, as never before participation of women, and that too from Scheduled Caste communities, had been witnessed in such large numbers. However, the result was disappointing, as the issue was rejected on two counts: first, that it was raised by Scheduled Caste women in a meeting dominated by the elites and second, that water was available to the people from the higher castes from other sources, including hand pumps, although they were not easily accessible to the poor and Scheduled Caste families.

The disappointing outcome prompted the women to start raising 10 per cent of the investment cost as their contribution for a hand pump in their own hamlet. Being a group of very poor women, they could shell out Rs. 2,000 from their savings. They went to the PHED office with their proposal, but were in for a rude shock when they learned that the installation of the hand pump, as estimated by the officials of the department, would require at least Rs. 60,000. The group resolved to put pressure again on the village panchayat, dominated by upper caste families, that they should contribute the remaining 50 per cent of the community contribution from the panchayat funds. This time they resorted to a different strategy and the group's members had a separate meeting with the women Sarpanch of the panchayat, who till then worked in the shadow of her husband.

This strategy had a telling effect as the Panchayat finally agreed, considering that it was its responsibility supply water to the Scheduled Caste hamlets. The proposal was prepared and submitted to the PHED and all formalities were completed at the earliest, but the department's clearance of the file took more than a year. It might have come to nothing if the group's leader, Balia Bai, president of the SHG and the village health committee and a Scheduled Caste and unlettered woman had not persisted together with the workers of Samarthan. Various kinds of pressure tactics were used to expedite the installation of the hand pump.

The group was ready to accept Rs. 50,000 or 10,000 less than the department's estimate, and manage the installation of the hand pump by themselves. They invited tenders from the contractors for drilling the bore well and checked the prices of hand pumps. This act shook up the PHED officials in Sehore. A local group was challenging the technical power of the department and ability to control such processes. Consequently, they started using technical hassles to delay the process. They sent across the message that the technical sanction would only be given when the drilling team was reimbursed using an inflated rate, i.e. at departmental rates which were higher than the market rates. Samarthan's team supported the group where they continued their struggle. There were many moments of frustration when the group wanted to give it up. Ultimately, the hand pump was sanctioned after a drawn out struggle lasting for more than a year.

The hand pump has been installed, benefitting 70 Scheduled Caste families, and its users are now collecting additional resources for the construction of a hand pump platform. Ramkali Bai, 55 years, expressed the response to the above process and its outcome in the following words: 'The only source for my livelihood comes from rearing goats for selling meat and milk to the villagers. I need to venture out to the nearby jungle early in the morning with the goats in tow and come back when it is dark. Drinking water for the family and the animals had to be arranged and that used to be hard, having to await my turn at the other hand pump. Now, with the installation of this hand pump near our hamlet, where one can fetch water any time of the day and without any discomfort after a day-long grind, things have become easier.'

On the flip side of the whole process, the PHED engineers are still asking for accounts, although they were presented in the gram sabha, a legitimate authority to approve all expenditure. The purpose is to bring more embarrassment to the committee.

The cases mentioned above clearly demonstrate the preparedness of the communities to manage their water supply by themselves and the unwillingness of the technical agencies and development administration to allow them to do so. The structural rigidities in the PHED and the district administration and the lack of mental preparedness to trust the abilities in the communities are primarily responsible for the slow implementation of development programmes by the local bodies and their local institutions. It is, therefore, pertinent to review the existing practices in one of the ongoing programmes of the Government of India, the Sector Reform Programme, which was designed to promote the involvement of the institutions for local self-governance.

BOTTLENECKS IN THE SECTOR REFORM PROJECT

The Sector Reform Programme is a pilot project of the Government of India which has adopted a clear strategy for community ownership of the local water supply by accepting demand-based requests from rural communities for water supply projects in which the processes of planning and implementation are controlled by the community and their local bodies.

Water supply programmes in India have been focussing on community participation for a few decades. However, such programmes have focussed mainly on community contributions in operation and maintenance. As water was the primary responsibility of the state, communities did not provide any hardware costs. This situation has now changed, as the communities are also asked to contribute to the capital cost of the projects.

In the district of Sehore, the Sector Reform Programme has been operational for the last two years. However, and as mentioned, the utilization of funds has been about one-third of the total amount available for this period. This strategy differs from the past, as previously the PHED did not delay project expenditures. As the guidelines provided by the central government were broad and the water supply departments of the states needed to convert them into operational details, it took more than expected time for the departments to respond. The departmental willingness to adopt the new approach was obviously low, as it demanded redesigning the role of the technical agency as a facilitator to help communities prepare their own plans for which they provided technical guidance in exploring alternative technical solutions. The institutional mechanisms for implementing the Sector Reform Project are depicted in Table 7.1.

Under the project, the district became the primary unit of operation and implementation. The Government of Madhya Pradesh decided to establish the District Level Coordination Committee (DLCC) at the zilla panchyat level. The committee was constituted under the chair of the zilla president, with membership from the officials of all the departments. It was expected that the committee would be responsible to clear proposals coming up from the villages for water supply and monitor their implementation.

In each block, a Block Level Coordination Committee (BLCC) was formed of which the chief executive officer (CEO) became the president, rather that the panchayat president, an elected representative. The members were various departmental heads located at the district level. This body was constituted to evaluate projects submitted in the villages and review their implementation. Bypassing democratically elected bodies may add efficiency, yet in the long term reduces degree of accountability of representatives for their voters.

In the same way, a structure at the panchayat level was proposed known as Project Level Coordination Committee (PLCC) where sarpanch became the president and panchayat members and development functionaries would be the members. This committee

Table 7.1: Operational Mechanism for the Sector Reform Project

Organization	Members	Responsibility
Apex Committee	President – Additional Chief Secretary, Secretary, Principal Secretary, PHED Members: Chief Secretary, Secretary-Panchayati Raj/Rural Development/ PHE/Health/Education /Finance/ Public Relation	Consultation and monitoring of strategy
Executive Body	President – Principal Secretary, PHED Members: Chief Engineer/Director – Rural Development/Panchayati Raj/ Education/Health/Social Welfare/ Information Broadcasting and Public Relation/NGO	Technical consultation and monitoring
District level	President – Zilla Panchayat President Members: Chief officers of all departments	Approval of proposals, implementation and monitoring
Block level Coordination Committee	President – Chief Executive Engineer Members: Block Development Officer Block-level Officers Development/Education/Health Executive Engineer/Women and Child Development Officer	Inspection of proposals, coordination and monitoring
Panchayat level Coordination Committee	President – Sarpanch Members – Representatives and village workers	Preparation of proposal implementation and monitoring
District Water and Sanitation Committee	President – Chief Executive Officer Secretary – Executive Engineer, PHE Members – Executive Engineer/District President/District Education Officer/ District Health Officer/Executive Engineer/DPRO/District Women and Children Development Officer/Child Development Officer/ICDS, Information and Public Relation and 3 NGOs.	Preparation of proposals, financial help through WATSAN Committee from the fund received from Government of India; Sign agreement with NGOs.

was expected to provide support in building micro-plans around water for submission to the appropriate body for sanction and implementation of the sanctioned plans. There is a very limited capacity within gram sabhas to build their micro-plans around water, especially taking into account the technical details required by the PHED to sanction projects.

It was presumed that the districts would be able to identify voluntary agencies which had expertise in the mobilization of the communities, as well as expertise in Participatory Rural Appraisals (PRA) to help villagers in developing micro-plans around water. The process could not be completed well in time, due to technical/procedural delays and the availability of a limited number of NGOs at the district level. A greater constraint was the attitudes of the district administration regarding NGO involvement. The potential of the NGOs was questioned and the authorities did not trust them to take up their intended roles. As a result, mobilization of the communities around the key objectives of the programme could not happen on a large scale.

The consequence of the district focus was that state level structures were not given enough emphasis. Within the given administrative mechanisms, district level official always look up to the state level officials for clear-cut directions. The intention that the districts would implement the project was meant make the clearance of community-planned local projects more efficient. However, it did not provide any alternative to deal with the existing centralized mechanisms and rigid hierarchies. The district authorities always looked up to the state level officials to provide directions and guidelines even for the issues that were to be settled at the local level.

Under the prevailing resistance to and shortage of NGOs, the PHED engineers in some of the districts decided to continue with the technical support and mobilization of the communities by themselves. The felt need for potable water in these districts was high due to the scarcity of enough and safe sources of drinking water. Communities were therefore willing to contribute up to 10 per cent to get a good water supply system, but they had limited capacities to plan the projects. There were complicated formats or no formats. The guidelines for preparing projects had not been clearly defined and the communities had not been informed about them. Furthermore, the capacity within the PHED was highly inadequate to reach out to a large number of villages and help them build comprehensive plans with precise technical details and estimates, especially in case of a piped water supply scheme or rainwater harvesting structures and watersheds for recharging groundwater.

The Sector Reform Programme expected that the villages would come up with a comprehensive plan for the supply of drinking water and the improvement of the groundwater situation, and that they would gradually implement the sanctioned plan based on their abilities to mobilize local contributions. Communities can, for example, initially mobilize contributions for a tubewell with a hand pump and later expand the well to a piped water supply scheme. Many of the villages have not been made aware of such an approach; therefore, in most cases there are only demands for either a hand pump or a piped water supply scheme. A comprehensive vision and long-term planning in the villages and small urban towns for water management is missing completely.

Voluntary organizations have been identified to support the gram sabhas in understanding programme guidelines, mobilizing household contributions and preparing and implementing plans for construction and operation, maintenance and management of water supplies and improved sanitation. There is a paucity of enough and capable voluntary agencies to cover such a large geographical area for support.

The procedures for contracting voluntary agencies are also cumbersome in terms of efficiency as it took more than two years to finalize the process for involving NGOs in the implementation of Sector Reform Programme. In the meantime, contractors interested to get contracts for hand pump installation or piped water supply scheme started mobilizing the villages they knew and supported them in making micro-plans for water supplies and water resources management. The interest of the contractors was primarily to get the contract and they were, therefore, willing to build schemes with much higher costs than actually required by building in the costs of 'speed money', as well as meeting part of the community contribution.

Procedural simplifications have now been proposed. Earlier, the chief engineer in the state capital signed the file for every single scheme. The new proposed structure suggests that the sub-engineer can sanction schemes up to Rs. 5 lakh on technical grounds and that the gram sabha can give the administrative sanction. The assistant engineer will technically approve schemes costing Rs. 5 to 10 lakh and the janpad panchayat will provide the administrative sanction. Schemes of more than Rs. 10 lakh will be technically sanctioned by the executive engineer and the district panchayat will provide administrative sanction. The change in decentralizing decision making at the district level and below will hasten the process of effective delivery of community-based projects. The spirit of decentralization of the water supply programme needs to percolate down to the administrative functioning, structures and procedures for the success of such community-based initiatives.

THE WAYS FORWARD

If self-government is to succeed, there is only one solution: to recognize and overcome constraints. The following are ways in which the programme could move forward:

Large-scale Campaign on Programme Objectives

There is a need to develop a large-scale campaign strategy as the Sector Reform Programme, which was piloted, in selected districts is being scaled up across the country as Swajaldhara. The experiences presented earlier have shown that the community members and representative of the panchayats are not fully aware of the programme and its procedures; therefore, wider dissemination of information in a 'Pulse Polio' campaign mode is essential. In an underdeveloped state such as Madhya Pradesh, there is a need to design and use methods of creative communication to reach out to the women and other less lettered groups in the communities. The Sector Reform Project suffered a great deal in terms of delay in initiating the project due to weak strategy for information dissemination. Methods of mass communication need to be used, such as radio and TV, to reach out to a large number of villages. There are examples of using radio to reach out to village populations with key messages of the programme developed by PRIA, Delhi, and other support organizations on local self-governance issues.

Reduced Control of the Line Agencies for Greater Effectiveness

It is an accepted fact that assurance of quality and adherence to the technical norms are prerequisites for any water supply system. However, the technical departments misuse the technical guidelines to retain power and control in their hand. There are cases under the Sector Reform Project where the department has centrally purchased equipments and materials at the district level on the pretext of quality control and economies of scale. However, this practice disempowers communities to check rates in the market and purchase the best-suited items of acceptable standards. Panchayat representatives should be able to get information about various types of hand pumps, pipes and engines at competitive prices and services. The PHED can take up the role of monitoring the quality of products which the private providers put on the market. The department can recognize official shops for communities to purchase items related with water supply. Incentives may be announced to those suppliers who are appreciated by the village bodies for their efficient services.

Strengthen Institutional Capacities and Performance-based Rewards

There is a need to recognize that the core competency of the PHED department is technical in nature. This is an essential requirement for a water and sanitation programme. The role of the PHED is to help communities identify locally appropriate technological options in water and sanitation. The engineers of PHED need to enhance their engineering abilities so that they can provide more quality services and see opportunities for their career enhancement. Staff who promote the strategies of the Sector Reform Programme and facilitate the process of community-based management of water and sanitation should be rewarded in the form of extra training, national and international exposure visits, promotions and increments. This will be helpful for changing the culture within the department for strengthening the institutional capacity for community-managed water supplies.

There is a need to sensitize the middle-level staff, which is closer to the communities and sits at the block level or in the district headquarter. Their sensitization as well as skill development on the relevance of governance, participation of women and participatory planning will be helpful to promote programmes such as the water sector reform. Staff of the PHED who move ahead with participatory management and develop innovative ways of relating with the panchayats to strengthen the decentralization process should be rewarded and promoted under a clear and formal policy of the department.

Simplification of Procedures and Greater Autonomy at the Local Level

The procedure for the preparation of micro-plans on water and sanitation is quite cumbersome. Moreover, technical sanctions as well as administrative sanctions required by the villagers make them vulnerable. In a scheme designed as a pro-people scheme, the community should be allowed to submit a proposal based on broad guidelines with simpler technical details. If they demonstrate that they have collected their contribution and are committed to mobilize more if required, there is a need to fix the responsibility of the PHED in specific terms. On submission of a proposal, the PHED should be responsible to convert it into a technical proposal in a specific period of say two weeks. The technical proposal must be sanctioned within say another two weeks and PHED should be responsible for the same. The villagers should not have to run around for the sanctioning. Any delays should cost the PHED a penalty, to be deposited in the village development fund. If the rates/estimates prepared by the PHED are higher than the market rates and the community agrees to get the work done at lower rates with equal standards and quality, the PHED should either accept this or deposit the surplus amount in the village development account on the completion of the scheme with the necessary certification by an independent panel of technical experts.

Strengthen Capacities on Micro-planning Technical Aspects and Women's Empowerment

There is a need to evolve simpler systems of micro-planning which the youths of the village can carry out by themselves. There are many examples of participatory planning developed by NGOs, which can be used to evolve more practical and simpler guidelines for planning in water and sanitation. Voluntary organizations will also provide training to the interested gram sabhas. The fees for paying NGOs and a sum to develop a proposal with sound technical consideration should be built into the project cost to be paid to the gram sabha/village, as part of the preparation of the application for the concerned administrative office.

Voluntary agencies undoubtedly have the required strengths for mobilizing people and facilitating processes which build the capacities of the panchayats and gram sabhas for micro-planning. NGOs can also disseminate knowledge about the programme and support the implementation of the water supply scheme. The scoping studies (Ch. 11), which have been taken up after a long time of implementation of the pilot project to determine the presence of various actors, especially NGOs, and their current capacities must be initiated right at the beginning of the project.

The department staff as well as NGOs need to build greater sensitivity and skill to promote equal participation of women and men in programmes. Many a times, even when participation of communities is large, the proportionate participation of women is ignored. Moreover, field-level workers need to know the difference between token and effective participation of women in water and sanitation programmes. The capacities of the staff need to be built for innovating techniques which provide greater opportunities for women to participate in overcoming social and other structural barriers. The staff also needs to build a strong value orientation to take position and see the value of women's involvement in water and sanitation.

Strengthen District/Block Level Panchayat Bodies for Greater Local Ownership

The executives, such as the chief executive officers and the collectors of the districts have a strong control over project implementation. Similarly, the PHED has retained its control though the provision of technical expertise. Local governance institutions need to be promoted and strengthened so that stakes of the effected representatives are strengthened. The zilla panchayat should become the centre of decision making for the water programme. The staff of the PHED should be attached to the zilla panchayats so that greater accountability of the staff towards the process of development may be ensured. The salaries of the line department should be released only on the approval of the District Water and Sanitation Committee, if the zilla and janpad representatives do not raise objections to the payment of salaries.

A sufficient allocation of funds is required to strengthen the offices of the district panchayats as well as build their capacities in programme management and governance functions. The offices of the janpad and zilla panchayats have inadequate infrastructure for efficient management of such an important programme; therefore, the management of programmes naturally is centralized in the PHED office or the office of the CEOs. There is a dearth of trained staff and absence of efficient technology such as computers and other equipments to make them efficient offices for supervising development programmes and improving the quality of governance at the local level.

EMERGING RESEARCH AGENDA

The experiences with the implementation of the Sector Reform Project with a people-centred approach on the one hand and enlarging the role of the institutions of local self-governance in the management of development on the other, have opened out enormous possibilities for research. Considering the fact that the Sector Reform Project will be scaled up with the purpose of keeping the PRIs at the centre, there is a need to undertake in-depth studies around the issues of local self-governance in relation to water and sanitation. The following research questions are identified in the context of institutional reform and grassroots governance:

Operational/Structural Issues

- How appropriate are the proposed institutions at the grassroots, especially the formation of committees? Do the water and sanitation committees have adequate powers, clarity of roles, and resources to fulfill their mandated objectives?
- Is participation of women and the poor adequately ensured or does it remain nominal? What are the processes adopted to enhance their participation?
- Are village panchayats, blocks or district-level panchayats and urban local bodies in small towns the most efficient and effective institutions for the implementation and monitoring of water and sanitation? What should be the best synergistic relationship of the variety of institutions with a potential for water and sanitation management?

- What are the best suited financial mechanisms to route the resources to PRIs in order to minimize control and unproductive delays, but with effective methods for their accountability?

Participation and Social Justice Issues

- Do self-help groups or other forms of organization enable women to collectively influence political decisions related to water management in their villages/blocks/districts?
- Do constitutional provisions of the gram sabha and a quorum for women and Dalits for the meetings significantly influence the quality of participation of women and Dalits on the issues of water and sanitation?
- To what extent can local governance bodies take up the issues of women/Dalits and poor in relation to equity in the distribution of water and what has been their role in decision making?
- Are norms of equity followed for attaining community contribution for capital or O&M costs? What are the levels of transparency and means of social audit adopted?

Comparative Analysis Issues

- Does any significant difference exist in the villages/peri-urban areas where there are examples of good governance compared with ineffective governance in relation to:
  - efficient management of water and sanitation;
  - cost recovery and sustenance of schemes; and
  - satisfaction levels of the women and other marginalized sections.
- Do differences in styles of leadership and systems and procedures have different impacts on the delivery of programmes in different types of villages/peri-urban areas?
- What are the necessary and sufficient conditions in different contexts for the co-existence of a diversity of institutions in a synergistic relationship on issues concerning water and sanitation?

The issues identified above are a suggestive list. They highlight the importance of research in a community-based water and sanitation programme. Capturing invaluable learning and understanding of processes' takes a backseat in an action-oriented programme. The challenges are primarily that a research agenda can be pursued and how this can be done.

At present, the monitoring systems of large-scale programmes as well as those of the NGOs are primarily designed either to inform targets and achievements or to assess performance of the field workers. It becomes, therefore, a controlling mechanism rather than a learning too'. At the designing stage of the monitoring system, research questions such as the above should be addressed and built into the system so that long-term process-oriented data may be generated around the research questions (van Wijk and Garcia, 2002). A team of research persons/coordinators should synthesize the data generated and bring out learning documents around various thematic issues.

Finally, there is a need to assign research issues to specialized agencies/research institutions and professional research consultants primarily for the purpose of comparative analysis as well as to have a more systematic handling of data and analysis. Sufficient resources need to be built in programme budgets so that an agenda of research can be pursued with sufficient attention and priority.

REFERENCES

Behar, Amitabh and Yogesh Kumar, 'Decentralisation in Madhya Pradesh, India: From Panchayati Raj to Gram Swaraj (1995 to 2001)', ODI, Working Paper 170, London: Overseas Development Institute, 2002.

Davis Jan, Gerry Carvey and Michael Wood, 'Developing and Managing Community Water Supplies', Oxfam Development Guideline No. 8. Oxford: OXFAM, 1993.

Government of India, 73rd Amendment Act, 1992, New Delhi: Ministry of Rural Development, 2004, *http://rural.nic.in/panch.htm*

Johnson, Craig, 'Decentralisation in India: Poverty, Politics and Panchayati Raj', Working Paper 199, London: Overseas Development Institute, 2003.

Knight, Barry, Hope Chugudu and Rajesh Tandon, *Reviving Democracy: Citizens at the Heart of Governance*, London: The Common Wealth Foundation, 2002.

Kumar, Yogesh, 'Building on the Panchayats: Using Jal Samitis in Uttar Pradesh', in Peter Bluent and D. Michael Warren (eds.), *Indigenous Organizations and Development*, London: Intermediate Technology Publications, 1996.

Kumar, Yogesh, Hasrat Arjjumend and R.N. Tiwari, 'Anatomy of Emerging Village Institutions and Its Implications in Decentralized Management of Development and Resources', *Proceedings of Foundation Day Seminar on Emerging Institutions for Decentralized Rural Development* organized by National Institute of Rural Development, Hyderabad, 2001.

Narain, Vishal, *Institutions, Technology and Water Control*, Wageningen: Wageningen University Water Resources Series, 2003.

PRIA, *Community Monitoring in Water and Sanitation Projects: A Facilitators Manual,* New Delhi: PRIA, 2002.

Rajiv Gandhi National Drinking Water Mission, 'Guidelines for Implementation of Rural Water Supply Programme', New Delhi: Ministry of Rural Development, 1999.

———, 'Finance Manual for Implementation of Sector Reform Pilot Projects', New Delhi: Ministry of Rural Development, 2001.

———, 'Guidelines on Sector Reform Pilot Project', New Delhi: Ministry of Rural Development, 2002.

Shetty, Salil, 'Development Project in Assessing Empowerment', Occasional Paper Series No. 3, New Delhi: Participatory Research in Asia, undated.

UNICEF, 'Jal Pradaya Evem Sampurna Grameen Swachhata Karyakram—Nai Ranneeti: Kriyanvan Margadarshika' (in Hindi), Bhopal: UNICEF, undated.

VANI, *State Panchayat Acts: A Critical Review,* New Delhi: Voluntary Action Network India, 1995.

Wijk, Christine van and Mariela Garcia, 'Having it Both Ways: Local Participatory Learning Informing Global Policy and Programme Management', in Cees Leeuwis and Rhiannon Pyburn (eds.), *Wheelbarrows Full of Frogs: Social Learning in Resource Management, International Research and Reflections*, Assen: van Gorcum, 2002, pp. 271-89, http://www.irc.nl/themes/gender

CHAPTER 8

Scaling Up Community-Managed Water and Sanitation in India: Pilot Projects

CHRISTINE SIJBESMA

INTRODUCTION

In the preceding decades, the state water supply engineering departments and water boards in India have greatly increased access to improved domestic water supplies for rural households. Results have been less positive for the reliable delivery of as per demand safe water. Progress in sanitation coverage and use has also lagged behind (Kolsky et al., 1999). Ample evidence exists from global research that more participatory planning and management of community water supplies and environmental sanitation gives better results in access for households within communities and functioning and use of the systems. More recently, quantitative studies confirmed that more, and more democratic participation in local planning decisions has a significant and positive relationship with better sustained and used community water supplies. Even stronger was the correlation with better management capabilities that are also more equitable for men and women and for the poor (Gross et al., 2001, van Wijk et al., 2002a). For more equitable access and better sustained systems, it is thus important to change from centrally planned, constructed and managed systems to local planning, implementation and management, with attention to equity for the women and the poor. Bilateral and multilateral cooperation has contributed to making forth these changes in India. This paper reports on two pilot projects that were scaled up to larger programmes, for water supply in north India and for sanitation in south India. The final section focusses on their relevance for the Indian sector reforms and the need for independent research for educative purposes.

RESEARCH ON COMMUNITY-MANAGED WATER SUPPLIES UNDER INDO-DUTCH COOPERATION

Research under the Indo–Dutch bilateral water and sanitation programme (1978–2003) has confirmed the importance of community planning and management for more sustainable and accessible water supplies. In Uttar Pradesh, Saraswat (1994) found that two community-managed piped gravity water supplies were functioning significantly better than a comparable government-managed scheme in the same area. The community-managed systems functioned reliably and performed admirably for 24 hours per day. The government-managed system was out of order for an average of one day per week and had intermittent supply during the other days. There were also considerable financial differences. The community-managed systems functioned at two-third to one-fourth of the standard operation and maintenance cost for the systems concerned. The costs in the government-managed water supply were over three times higher (Table 8.1). In one community-managed scheme, young women and men did most of the maintenance.

Other studies confirmed the importance of user participation in planning decisions. In Andhra Pradesh, the utility built piped water supplies scheme was implemented without participation of the future users in choosing the type of system, the local designs, and the local operation, maintenance, management and financing arrangements. After completion, they handed over the systems to the local government for operation and maintenance. The resulting services had low

Table 8.1: Functioning and O&M Costs of Three Rural Water Supplies by Type of Management

Type of management of water supply	Name and year of commissioning	Functioning	Standard O&M cost p.p.	Actual O&M cost p.p.
Community-managed	Talli Kheri Khurd (1991)	7 days/week 18 hrs/day	INR 35.74	INR 8.82
	Mohammad Pur Kemri (1992)	7 days/week 24 hrs/day	INR 26.70	INR 16.00
Utility-managed	Mal Devta (1993)	6 days/week 24 hrs/day	INR 12.90	INR 44.00

Source: Saraswat, 1994.

levels of access for the poor and their functioning and cost-recovery were unsatisfactory. The users nevertheless preferred that their local government operated the systems. Only 13 per cent users wanted the State agencies to take over the management (Job and Shastry, 1991).

Full participation of both sexes, and not just the men, in decision planning lead to more equal access for the poor. Partial participation had only partially positive results. Both findings were from studies in Kerala, where at that time, and in contrast to the states of Uttar and Andhra Pradesh, none of the rural water supplies was community-managed. However, participation of, in particular, community women in the selection of stand post sites in Danish and Dutch-supported rural water projects improved distribution of public taps within the communities and raised their actual use (Zachariah, 1987; SEUF, 1994 and Fig. 8.1).

A second Kerala study confirmed that influence of users, especially of women, on site selection led to better distribution and access of community water points for low-income groups. Higher and middle income households usually had their own private connections. However, it was also found that only half of the households using community taps did so during the wet season and 56 per cent during the dry season. The reason was the poor functioning of the government-operated schemes (Kurup and Wanikumar, 1997).

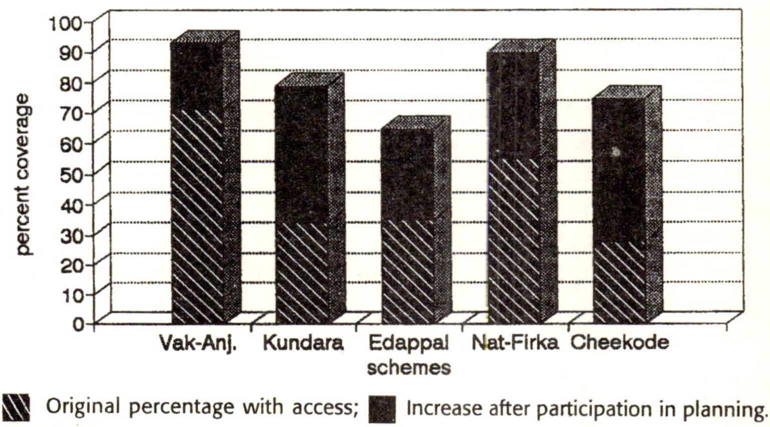

Fig. 8.1: Increase in Percentage of People Living within 250 m. of a Public Stand Post After Participatory Site Selection with Women and Men in Five Piped Water Schemes

Table 8.2: Percentage Recovery of O&M Costs in Indo-Dutch Assisted Piped Water Supplies in Three States as Compared to Average Cost Recovery

State	Scheme	% cost recovery in Indo-Dutch schemes	% cost-recovery in all piped schemes
Gujarat	Santalpur	2	1.5
	Lathi Lilya	7.4	
	Sami Harij	20	
Kerala	Kondotti	66	21.4
	Nattika Firka	25	
	Mala	9	
Uttar Pradesh	Sub-project I	25.6	No information
	Sub-project IV	20-25	

Source: Kurup et al., 1996

Community-based organizations and local government bodies could only replace washers and had to report all other problems of functioning to the utility. They had then to wait for the utility to act and could not bring in authorized repair workers themselves (Pillai and Menon, 1995). There is further evidence to suggest that when users have some say in the planning and operation of the schemes, the percentage of bill payment is somewhat higher (Kurup et al., 1996 and Table 8.2).

In water supplies implemented by the State agencies only, access for the poor and the actual use of the improved systems are seldom investigated. The utility and governments simply assume that when a community gets water supply, the whole of the population is served. In reality, this is not necessarily the case because in utility-planned water supplies there is no influence of, and accountability to, of the common women and men community members on how the available numbers of community taps are to be distributed over the local neighbourhoods. As a result, communal taps may only be located along the main roads while the backlanes and outlying hamlets get no service.

EXPERIENCES WITH RURAL SANITATION

In comparison with rural drinking water supplies, work on rural sanitation has been limited. Community sanitation has also been researched less on sustainability and use and the relationship with participatory and gender and class specific planning and management (Kolsky et al., 1999). This was not different in the Indo–Dutch water and sanitation projects where, with the exception of Kerala, the number of communities with work on sanitation was much smaller than for water supply (Ministry of Foreign Affairs, 1992 and Table 8.3). The adopted strategy was that field staff from a local NGO (in Gujarat, and later Andhra Pradesh) or a temporary and Dutch-financed Project unit (in Karnataka, Kerala and Uttar Pradesh) provided highly subsidized and sometimes fully subsidized latrines to a small number of households below the poverty line.

The research showed that with intensive social support for promotion of health education and monitoring, most household members used the latrines for human excreta disposal. A comparative study in Uttar Pradesh between the intensive Indo-Dutch projects and a state government project in the same area found that though the latter had a lower unit cost per installed latrine, it was not a success with the users. The intensive approach thus bore fruit, but the high subsidies and the employment of externally paid staff made its application on a large scale unsustainable (Woersem et al., 1992; Schaik et al., 1998).

The only state where the Indo–Dutch programme developed a large-scale sanitation approach was Kerala (Table 8.3). The Socio-Economic Unit first tried out three different approaches in a small-scale experiment. The strategies tested were: (i) direct implementation by their own staff; (ii) implementation by local NGOs; and (iii) implementation by the Panchayat in cooperation with locally chosen user committees. Comparison of the costs and outcomes of the three

Table 8.3: Latrines Constructed in Indo–Dutch Projects in Four States 1987–91

State	Planned coverage (households)	Realized	Planned coverage (institutions)	Realized	Community latrines constructed
Andhra Pradesh	14,500	354	472	22	1
Gujarat	–	–	–	–	–
Kerala	12,000	6,500	–	30	1
Uttar Pradesh	3,591	1,277	–	–	–
Total	30,091	8,126	472	52	2

Source: Operations Review Unit, 1994.

strategies showed that the first approach had the best results, but was also the most costly. The results of the second approach differed per NGO. The third approach had the best match between cost and results, and was, therefore, adopted for replication on a larger scale.

Characteristic for the strategy were the participatory planning and management of community sanitation interventions and the high involvement of women in planning and management and as paid latrine masons. The locally formed ward water and sanitation committees and the local government planned, implemented and managed community sanitation together. Each ward committee had seven members, including at least three women. The women were not figureheads, but participated in local decision-making and management. Many of them have now been elected for local government bodies. The ward committees chose the households whose poverty qualified them for a subsidized latrine. They printed their choices (lists were, for example, pinned to trees) and community members could both oppose and change decisions.

Between 1992 and 1997, external latrine subsidies from Dutch funds fell from 80 per cent to 15 per cent. Instead, latrine subsidies were increasingly financed through a combination of local government funds and voluntary contributions from local charities and neighbours. Contracts of the Panchayats with the project defined the contribution from panchayat and households, the responsibilities of the parties, the donor share (managed by the SEUF), the unit costs, fund flow, payment arrangements, accountability and the open-ended duration of the support, until the time that all poor households had a latrine. In 1995, the average cost of the latrines was Rs. 2,250–2,500 per latrine, including 6–9 per cent for social and administrative support from the NGO. These costs compared favourably with the cost of the latrines in Uttar Pradesh which were already Rs. 6,440 in 1991, including 20 per cent government overhead costs. Better-off households could join the programme at their own costs. Each panchayat could also join in a school sanitation programme.

Latrine construction was only step 9 to 11 in a 13-step cycle. Part of the process was that male and female household heads participated in three educative sessions—on health, hygiene, and operation and maintenance. After construction, the ward committees visited each household three times at increasing time intervals to see whether all household members used the latrines. They also monitored hygiene, hand washing and proper operation. Internal project research in 11 panchayats showed that on an average 96 per cent of the latrines were in use as toilets. Excreta disposal of children under five and hand washing could still be improved (Kurup et al., 1996).

The results were encouraging. Between 1991 and 1996, 58 panchayats with a total population of 1.4 million people joined the programme. Together, ward committees and Panchayats helped 85,000 households, of which 75,000 were below the poverty line, install a sanitary latrine. The supporting NGO increasingly trained poor women as masons. In Kerala, as elsewhere in India, masons are men while women as mason helpers do the unskilled manual work. They work on temporary contracts and are often treated badly and sexually abused. When the migration of craftsmen to the Gulf countries caused a shortage, the NGO began to train groups of women mason helpers to become skilled latrine block makers and builders. The training centre has now become the autonomous Jeevapoorna Women Mason's Society. It expanded training to five districts. There are over 1,200 trained women masons and 250 have developed into fully skilled construction workers who work in the housing industry and have their own cooperative (van Wijk et al., 2002b). The training and group work built up the women's self-confidence and endowed them with skills to solve problems together. The shift from helper to mason has doubled their income and enhanced their status and (self) respect (Raghavan, 2000).

SCALING UP TO DISTRICT LEVEL AND BEYOND

Projects supported by external loans or grant, such as the one described earlier, provided professionals in Indian NGOs and utilities with opportunities to try out innovative approaches for which state programmes and policies did not provide space. These experiments started small but some grew to include the district and beyond. Two of them are analysed below. The 'Clean Kerala' programme evolved from the Danish and Dutch supported project described earlier. The Swajal Project in Uttar Pradesh in northern India was supported by the World Bank. It focussed mainly on community-managed rural water supply, although some sanitation and hygiene promotion were included. Another scaled up project for rural sanitation, in West Bengal, was supported by UNICEF. This is similar to the project in Kerala in the sense that a local NGO played a central role. The approach is, however, more geared towards marketing of low-cost latrines directly to rural households, rather than on local government and ward committees investigating local conditions and making and implementing local community action plans (Kolsky et al., 1999).

SANITATION IN KERALA

In 1991, 5.5 million households in Kerala had no sanitary latrine. Of them, 85 per cent were poor. The State sanitation programme was not popular and did not succeed in closing the sanitation gap. Due to the annual population growth, about half of the poor households continued to live without latrines. The bilaterally supported sanitation programme gave good results, but its scope was insufficient to make more than limited inroads.

The state sanitation policy and programme then changed through a combination of pressures from the unserved poor and state-planned reforms. When unserved populations in panchayats neighbouring those with Indo–Dutch–Danish projects saw the progress and quality of community-managed sanitation, they put pressure on their local governments to change from state-managed to panchayat-managed sanitation interventions. In 1997, 5 of the 14 district panchayats launched their own panchayat-managed programmes for total sanitation. In 1998, this became a state-wide programme of 'Clean Kerala'.

In the same year, the People's Planning Campaign took place in 990 panchayats throughout Kerala. In this campaign, women and men formulated their development priorities in public meetings and identified, among others, 1,793 sanitation projects with a total estimated cost of Rs. 303 million (US $4,50,000). To meet these people's formulated priorities, the state government devolved 35–40 per cent of its annual plan funds to the panchayats between 1997 and 2000. A Task Force on Sanitation formulated a new state strategy for sanitation. This strategy reduced the state's subsidy and allowed households to choose their own latrine types. It authorized that local governments, Ward Water and Sanitation Committees and local Neighbourhood Committees plan, implement and manage the community sanitation projects. SEUF became a member of the Task Force and shifted to training.

During the first three years, panchayats and households together built 4,13,000 latrines, more than three times the 1,25,000 latrines built during Kerala's Eighth Five Year Plan. The People's Plan which underlies the programme is under threat, however. The Congress-led coalition defeated the ruling leftist party in the state elections in May 2001 and lowered the allocation of Plan funds to the panchayats by 16.4 per cent. It also granted Rs. 2,50,000 to each member of the legislative assembly to spend in their constituencies. It has changed the composition and decision-making rules of the Task Force in such a way that the influence of government officials has increased. The position of coordinator at the block and district level has been removed. This position is filled predominantly by representatives from civic society. Regulations which ensured women's representation in decision-making on all development projects have been removed, except for the so-called women's projects. Women's Self Help Groups that get Plan Funds can no longer have members who according to state government criteria are 'above the poverty line'. This new rule has suddenly excluded all women who work 10 days or more per month as agricultural labourers, as this makes them qualify as 'above poverty line. It has put an abrupt end to many existing groups and to the formation of new ones (Mohanakumar, 2002).

Water Supply and Sanitation in Uttar Pradesh

The Swajal Project for community-managed water and sanitation took place in the part of the state of Uttar Pradesh in north India where water is scarcest so that both need and demand would be high. Its budget was US $71 million. It was financed through an 84 per cent World Bank loan and a 6 per cent State grant. The aim was to enable community women and men to plan, construct and manage the kind of water supply and sanitation systems that they wanted and could sustain. The project covered some 1,200 rural communities, 1 per cent of the total in the state. Locally recruited NGOs, consultancy firms and legally recognized community groups became the project catalysts. As Support Organizations (SO), they assisted the villagers in initiation, planning and implementation of local water, sanitation and hygiene projects and trained them for local management. Eligibility conditions were legal registration for a minimum of three years, at least three years' experience in the water sector or in general community development, successful completion of minimally one water and sanitation project with participation and women's involvement, presence of social and engineering staff and evidence of sound financial management. The project management ranked candidate SOs on a 0-100 scale and the Project Committee made the final choice. This committee consisted of 15 high ranking government officials and four members who represented the field: one Community Development Officer and three NGO representatives.

The SO teams visited communities which met the national criteria of a poor water supply and/or health. If they were interested, the SOs prepared a feasibility report. The project staff validated the reports and chose the ones which scored best on need, demand, and technical and institutional feasibility. The SOs then helped the selected communities prepare village action plans. A plan ideally covered a new water supply with arrangements for maintenance and financing, sanitation improvement, hygiene promotion, catchment area protection, a women's income generating project and a women's non-formal education project. The communities had to contribute 10 per cent of the investment costs of the water supply as a sign of demand and pledge to bear the costs of keeping the service operational. They opened a bank account and formed water and sanitation committees.

The SOs monitored which decisions were discussed in the community meetings, what percentages of the villagers attended and how many of them were women. Women participated first in separate meetings at the neighbourhood level. Here they prepared their own sub-plans on income generation, hygiene campaigns (considered a women's only subject) and non-formal education. Minimally 30 per cent of the committee members had to be women and 20 per cent had to belong to marginal social groups.

New in Swajal was the aim of establishing autonomous, community-managed water services and water-related development. The water supplies would be maintained, managed and financed by local committees that had been chosen by consensus for their specific tasks and had received training. Planning was given more time than construction and was made more participatory, flexible and gender- and poverty-sensitive. The communities and user households could make informed choices on technologies and designs. Separate meetings for women at the neighbourhood level gave poor women better access to information and helped women organize around common interests.

To make the process and benefits more equitable for poor people, Swajal stipulated that planned services had to provide access to all households, that committees had to have quota for poor members and that those households who wanted a higher service level had to pay more. Financing, accountability and administration differed greatly from the approach in government programmes. In line with project principles in the private sector, SOs and communities had to compete for funds based on published rules. Adherence to these rules was controlled through an internal peer control system. SOs were accountable to the communities as well as the Swajal management. Direct transfer of funds to the community project account, transparency and village peer control (budgets and costs had to be made known to the full committee) were introduced to lower misuse of funds. The project administration no longer directly implemented the community projects, but enabled the Panchayats to plan and implement their own services.

In other respects, top-down decisions and inflexibility continued. The project prescribed the water tariffs. These had to be monthly and a minimal amount of Rs. 30 (US $0.75) for a private tap and Rs. 10 for public tap users was agreed upon. Outsiders also fixed the duration and location of community projects. The cycle of 33 months which the project had decided on made it hard for individual communities to proceed at their own speed. The SOs determined project locations by deciding which communities they would visit. And since the SOs needed to win contracts for community projects they may have favoured villages with higher demands and potentials. Under a similar policy in Colombia, the most disadvantaged communities with the lowest technical and economic opportunities had remained unserved when visited 10 years later (van Wijk and Heijnen, 1981). Decisions to allocate community projects were still also made from the top. Although there were rules, and internal control and decisions were accounted for in letters to the SOs, allocation decisions were made in internal project meetings and no representatives of the communities and SOs were allowed to attend.

The more equitable financing model has still disadvantaged the rural poor. The adopted policy, which is continued under the national sector reform, was that communities paid 10 per cent of the investment cost of the water supply. When a community opted for a piped water supply with house connections, the benefitting house-holds therefore paid more than when the preferred choice was for public taps or hand pumps. However, the other 90 per cent of the investment costs then also constituted a much larger amount. In consequence, the higher the chosen technology and service level, the fewer unserved communities could be served with the available project funds. The case in Box 8.1 illustrates the macro-economic bias of the investment financing system.

The financing system would only have been equitable if the private connection owners would have paid the full incremental cost of their higher service level. It is further not clear whether the SOs helped communities set up more equitable and locally adapted systems for labour contributions and payments for public taps. Also not clear is whether communities were encouraged to go for upgrading the existing water supplies rather than building a totally new water supply instead of or next to the already existing services.

Box 8.1: Some for All or More for Some? In-built Financing Bias for Poor People

In Laxmipur, in Dehradun district at the foot of the Himalaya, the inhabitants had a choice between three technology options: individual rainwater tanks, six hand pumps or a piped water supply with house connections and standpipes. They rejected rainwater storage as they did not like the idea of storing drinking water for six months. The cost for six hand pumps was Rs. 3,00,000 and the cost for a piped system was Rs. 26,00,000. The village had to make a down payment of 1 per cent for the piped system and could contribute the other 9 per cent in labour for digging drenches. For the hand pumps they had to pay the full 10 per cent in cash. The economics were clear. The piped system required a down payment of Rs. 26,000 and provided the chance of water within the house; hand pumps required Rs. 30,000 and meant water points were shared and water still had to be carried. Not surprisingly, the village chose to dig and got a system nearly ten times more expensive than the hand pumps.

No information could be found on the effects of the community projects on the overall water resources in the water catchment areas. Several projects in the same catchment area and more and larger groups of people using the same water resources for different and often competitive uses may have led to increased problems with water resources management.

Finally, questions can be posed about the project's gender strategy as it mixed women's welfare, poverty alleviation, project efficiency, and project effectiveness objectives. The hygiene promotion component reflected a typical welfare strategy. Although the project recognized that in sanitation and hygiene women are key actors and transmitters of knowledge, the approach placed the burden health and hygiene responsibilities on women only. The gender division of labour and decision-making between women and men was not questioned. There was no mention of men's practices, responsibilities and decision-making on sanitation, hygiene and health. Extra work in the 'healthy homes' surveys and the cleaning up campaigns was expected from the women. No link was made with the time analysis exercises that had been done with them in the earlier pre-planning stage and which had shown that women already worked longer hours than men. The planned income generation projects, which were typical for a women-in-development approach, were in practice seldom successful as SOs lacked expertise and experience in creating financially viable micro-enterprises with women. Nor was it clear which socio-economic class of women participated in and benefitted from the economic projects and how this affected women's positions in the households and the community. Iyer (1998, 1999) reported that the new paradigm was effective in terms of integrating women and the poor in water supply management. During the first batch of community projects, committee membership of women (42 per cent) and people from Scheduled Castes and Tribes (35 per cent) surpassed the project quota. However, the women also contributed most of the voluntary work. The project did not compare the voluntary work and benefits of the women and the poor with those of men and the better-off to see whether they were equitably divided. From the project's information it cannot be excluded that the less advantaged made more contributions, while the most advantaged reaped more benefits.

From the above it can be concluded that for the further scaling up of community-managed water supplies and sanitation, much could be learned from the more in-depth analysis of experiences with these interesting programmes. Until now, such in-depth analysis has not taken place. The Indo–Dutch Programme on Alternatives in Development (IDPAD), in which Indian and Dutch researchers jointly undertake research, offers a framework for formulating and implementing such a study. In the following section, some research questions are raised and research methods discussed.

RELEVANCE FOR THE INDIAN DECENTRALISATION POLICY

The findings from research and pilots summarized here are important in the light of the Indian policy reforms on the decentralization of basic community services to local government. Under the 73rd and 74th constitutional amendments, the Indian government reinstituted the local government system in 1992. The reforms gave the locally elected bodies the power to act directly on 29 development subjects including community water supply and sanitation. Progress with the implementation of this policy has varied between the states (Ministry of Rural Areas and Development, 1999). The great challenge for water supply and sanitation is to implement the policy on a scale that goes from a small number of communities to whole districts and beyond, with the same results for universal access, sustained functioning and use, and gender and social equity.

To implement decentralized water supply and sanitation, the Rajiv Gandhi Drinking Water Mission has launched two Sector Reform Programmes. The Accelerated Rural Water Supply Programme (ARWSP) has been revamped from a target-based, supply-driven programme to a demand-responsive programme where users get the service they want and are willing to pay for. Twenty per cent of the annual outlay of the ARWSP has been earmarked for allocation to states that want to institutionalize community-managed rural water supplies. The objective of the reform is to have financially and environmentally sustainable rural water supply systems through management at the lowest appropriate level. The reform provides a long-term incentive to the Indian states, relieving them of the current burden of recurrent costs and rehabilitation of systems. To qualify for a share in these funds, the states have to replace their top-down, supply-driven delivery of rural water supplies by a demand-responsive and adaptable approach. Under this approach, and if wanted with the help of NGOs, they are to assist the villagers to plan for, install, maintain and run their own water supply services. The community management includes all technical, financial and administrative tasks involved in keeping the services going and providing water to all community households. The communities must partially share the capital costs (10 per cent), either in cash or kind or both, and take full responsibility for operation and maintenance.

Sixty-three districts from all over India entered the reform programme on a pilot basis. Activities included the preparation of comprehensive action plans by states and districts based on comprehensive village water and sanitation planning; some adoption of participatory methods; human resource development aimed at empowering the Panchayati Raj Institutions (PRI) and local communities; information, education and communication (IEC) activities related to hardware (technologies, designs) and software aspects (community participation and gender); monitoring and evaluation; and special attention to water quality, source sustainability and the provision of drinking water in rural schools.

The Centrally Sponsored Rural Sanitation Programme (CSRSP) has also been restructured. Its new strategy aims at accelerating the coverage of the rural population to 50 per cent during the Ninth Plan by stimulating demand for latrines through awareness creation and health education. Users are to be given a choice of sanitation technologies of different types and costs to suit local variations in demands, payment capacities and physical and cultural conditions. In addition, the programme will provide schools in rural areas with sanitation facilities. Intensive IEC activities are to promote sanitation as a means to achieving a better quality of life.

As with water supply, the sanitation reform was planned to be community-led and people-centred. A demand-driven approach was adopted with stress on awareness building and meeting the demand with alternate delivery mechanisms: sanitation production centres producing slabs and blocks, rural sanitary marts where consumers can buy materials, and (re)trained village masons. The national reforms required state engineering departments to restructure and move towards decentralized models of service delivery with the PRIs, non-profit organizations, civil society organizations, and so on. The policy further foresaw the gradual phasing out of subsidies for individual latrine units. More than 115 districts were designated as 'sanitation districts'.

For both sanitation and water supply, a few states and districts have fully entered the new programmes. Some have completed policy frameworks and/or started with internal capacity building; others are just beginning. A minority has devolved power and/or funding. Meanwhile, the central level has already sent a large share of the financial resources. Operationalization, organizational reforms and the use of national funds by agencies other than those of the state in this gradual devolution to district and panchayat have remained major challenges. The second case study will show the effects of the late attention given to these important conditions for policy implementation.

RESEARCH ON SCALING UP FOR NATIONAL POLICIES AND PROGRAMMES

So far, no in-depth research of the scaled up pilot projects has been carried out, although there have been a number of smaller investigations. A participatory evaluation in 10 panchayats in Kerala compared the relationships between participation, gender and poverty processes and the sustainability and use of rural water supplies and community-managed sanitation. The study was part of a global evaluation of 88 community-managed services on the linkages between sustainability and use of water and sanitation and demand, gender and poverty approaches (Gross et al., 2001). In Kerala, the results for sanitation were significantly better than for the less participatory rural water supply services (WSP, unpublished data).

A gap in the scaling up of community management of water supply and sanitation in India is that the experience with larger scale implementation which were gained over the last five years in various parts of the country have not been systematically analysed. In three parts of India, Uttar Pradesh in the north, West Bengal in the east and Kerala in the south, non-governmental support organizations have helped Panchayats and community-based organizations to plan, implement and manage improved water supplies and/or sanitation at and above district level. Since the Indian government is now implementing a policy of decentralized governance, it would be valuable to investigate in the field the effectiveness and costs of the strategies used in these larger-scale approaches. Such research would also be quite useful in a global context as governments in many other countries who have similar policies and face problems of implementation of decentralized water supply and sanitation may learn from the research generated by the Indian endeavour.

Questions that could be the basis for such research relate especially to the kind of support given to the communities, the effectiveness of that support, and the factors that might explain the differences in degrees of success in processes and results. Some typical questions would be:

- How effective have SOs been in enabling local communities to plan, implement and manage their own water supply and/or sanitation projects?
- What is the quality of the established facilities and services and the equality of processes and results with regard to gender and poverty?
- Which community and agency factors may explain why some communities and SOs perform better than others?
- How much did community-managed water supply and sanitation cost in terms of direct costs (investment and operations) and costs of support? How do these costs compare with those of utility-managed systems?
- What have been the experiences and reactions of districts and line departments? Have any continued or replicated the projects or adopted more facilitating approaches? To what extent have communities been able to call in technical and other expertise from others (NGOs, private sector)?

Experiences with this kind of research exist in India. Some of them have been reported in this article. Almost all these studies have been carried out as non-participatory studies, however. Women and men community members and members of panchayats, water and sanitation committees and representatives of the support and project agencies have not been involved. This non-participatory character of the research has lowered opportunities for ownership and use of the results by exactly those parties on which the application of the learning depends. Hence, it is recommended that any proposal for research on community-managed water supply and sanitation includes plan for a participatory approach. In participatory research the different stakeholders in the communities and agencies participate in the research along with external researchers from India and the Netherlands.

REFERENCES

Gross, Bruce, Christine van Wijk, and Nilanjana Mukherjee, 'Linking Sustainability with Demand, Gender and Poverty: A Study in Community-Managed Water Supply Projects in 15 Countries', Washington: World Bank Water and Sanitation Program, 2001.

Iyer, Parameswaran, 'Uttar Pradesh State, India: The Swajal Project, Experiences with Implementing a Demand-responsive Approach', paper presented at the Community Water Supply and Sanitation Conference, 5-8 May 1998, Washington D.C.: World Bank, http://www.wsp.org/English/ Conference/case/india.html

———, 'Mechanisms for Sustainability in a Supply-Driven Environment', *Waterlines*, 18 (1), 1999, pp. 25–8.

Job, P.J. and D.S. Shastry, 'Village-level Water Supply Management: Study on Nalgonda Mandal, Nalgonda District', Hyderabad: Netherlands-Assisted Project Office and Panchayati Raj Engineering Department, 1991.

Kolsky, P., E. Baumann, R. Bhatia, J. Chilton and C. van Wijk, 'Evaluation of UNICEF Water and Environmental Sanitation Activities in India 1966–1998', New Delhi: UNICEF, 1999.

Kurup, A.M. and A.S. Wanikumar, 'A Water Use Survey of the Six Netherlands-assisted Water Supply Schemes: Changing Pattern of Water Use in Rural Kerala', Thiruvananthapuram: Society for Psycho-social Research and Rehabilitation, 1997.

Kurup, K.B. et al., 'Of Flows and Flush', synthesis paper presented at the National Workshop on Operation and Maintenance of Rural Water Supply and Sanitation Systems, New Delhi, 25–7 September 1996.

Ministry of Foreign Affairs, 'Latrine Projects in the Indo-Dutch Rural Water Supply and Sanitation Programme: A Discussion Paper', The Hague: Ministry of Foreign Affairs, Directorate General International Co-operation, South Asia Country Section, 1992.

Ministry of Rural Areas and Employment, 'Panchayati Raj Institutions in

India: States Doing Well/Doing Not So Well With Reference to Certain Matters', New Delhi: Government of India, 1999.

Mohanakumar, S., 'From People's Plan to Plan Sans People', *Economic and Political Weekly*, 20 April 2002, pp. 1492–7.

Operations Review Unit, 'India: Evaluation of the Netherlands Development Programme with India, 1980–1992', The Hague: Ministry of Foreign Affairs, Operations Review Unit, 1994.

Pillai, S.R. and T.A. Menon, 'Operation and Maintenance of Rural Water Supply Schemes of Kerala Water Authority: A Study on the Non-technical and Managerial Aspects of Edappal, Mala and Choondal Schemes', Thiruvananthapuram: Institute of Management in Government, 1995.

Raghavan, Rajiv, 'Building the Balance: Stories on Water, Sanitation and Gender Equity from Kerala, India', Delft: IRC International Water and Sanitation Centre, 2000.

Saraswat, R.D., 'Evaluation of Functioning, Quality Parameters and Possibility of Community Management in Gravity-fed Rural Water Supply Schemes in Garhwal, Uttar Pradesh, India', M.Sc. thesis, Delft: IHE, 1994.

Schaik, H.P.J. van, P. Vyasulu, K.M. Namboodiri, 'Indo-Dutch Cooperation Programme in Rural Water Supply and Sanitation, Uttar Pradesh, India. Performance Assessment and Future Planning', Bilthoven: RIVM, 1998.

SEUF, 'Locating Public Standposts with the Community: The Impact of Site Selection Procedures on Water Schemes in Kerala', Trivandrum: Socio-Economic Units, 1994.

Wijk, Christine van and Han Heijnen, 'Report on the Slow Sand Filtration Demonstration Project in Colombia', The Hague: IRC International Water and Sanitation Centre, 1981.

Wijk, Christine van, Prathap K. Reddy and Thresiamma Mathew, 'Water Supply, Sanitation and Rural Poverty Reduction in Gujarat and Kerala States', The Hague: Institute of Social Studies, 2002a.

Wijk, Christine van, Kumala Sari, Nina Shatifan, Ruth Walujan, Ishani Mukherjee, Richard Hopkins, 'Flores Revisited: Sustainability, Hygiene and Use of Community-managed Water Supply and Sanitation and the Relationships with Project Approaches and Rules', Jakarta: Water and Sanitation Program, Delft: IRC, 2002b.

Woersem, B. van, A.R. Manuel, B. Kakkar 'Indo-Dutch Rural Water Supply and Sanitation Projects, Uttar Pradesh, India', Report of the 1992 Evaluation Mission, Breukelen: Aqua, 1992.

Zachariah, Elizabeth, 'Water Utilization Study on Existing Water Supply Schemes in Danida-selected Project Areas', unpublished report, 1987.

CHAPTER 9

Capacity Development for Reform in India's Water Supply and Sanitation: A Case Study

KATHLEEN SHORDT

INTRODUCTION

Community management and decentralization are two sides of a coin. They can only be scaled up with quality if capacity is in place. This paper describes an attempt at an innovative programme that initiated district capacity development to support the national water and sanitation sector reforms of India in 2002. The programme was undertaken in partnership with the Ministry of Rural Development of the Government of India, UNICEF–India and governmental and non-governmental stakeholders within districts. It was facilitated by a core group composed of Indian professionals working together with the staff of the International Water and Sanitation Centre (IRC), and the Water, Engineering and Development Centre (WEDC) of Loughborough University in the UK. The paper examines the capacity development effort, processes and outputs. The final section focuses on lessons learned that would hopefully be relevant to other similar efforts.[1]

CONCEPTS

Reform of the water and sanitation sector in India is meant to lead to decentralization, community management, improved water and sanitation services with increasing demand for household sanitation. Key sector stakeholders recognize that in order to reach the objectives of the sector reform, the capacity of those working at the many levels in the states needs to be enhanced.

Before the specific details of the programme are discussed, the conceptual underpinnings of capacity development programme and of sector reform are presented in this section.

Decentralization: Decentralization refers to the transfer of practices and responsibilities of governance closer to the citizenry. It involves shifting functions and work, administration as well as decision-making authority, to communities or other groups such as private institutions or non-governmental organizations. In this sense, decentralization goes beyond requiring communities to contribute to construction or take responsibility for operation and maintenance of water services.

Community management: The central meaning of community management is control, rather than carrying out work such as operation and maintenance. Control includes decision-making powers that put the community in charge, in other words, real management. Community refers to all people or to representatives of all major groups . . . different classes, castes, ages, men and women. Representatives should be endorsed by the majority and genuinely representative of their groups and not just of a community minority. If only a few richer families control a system, that system is unlikely to serve the needs and interests of the entire community (Schouten and Moriarty, 2003).

> Community management builds from the bottom up, while decentralization typically comes from the top down. Where they meet is somewhere in the middle, typically around the level of district or municipal government. Both community management and decentralization will still take a long time to mature, but they cannot do without each other. (Schouten and Moriarty, 2003, p. 132)

Scaling up community management: Scaling up means that good experience, models of success and experienced people are brought in to adapt and extend strategies, with quality, to other areas (IRC, 2002). While scaling up usually requires expanding the coverage internally (for example, covering all communities in a district) or laterally (expanding to other districts), it requires far more than construction.

Scaling up of community management requires backstopping the new community capacities almost indefinitely, until the age of retirement, to bring legal accountability to financial management, to facilitate disagreements and resolve conflicts, to ensure the vulnerable groups are not excluded. In a nation the size of India, this is quite obviously a monumental challenge.

Capacity development: In this programme, capacity development was seen as more than training, focussing on three critical issues:

- Attitudes and motivation ('We want to do it'.)
- Skills, knowledge and experience ('We know how and can do it'.)
- The enabling environment ('We are able to do it'.)

Participants: Whose capacities are to be built? Capacity development in the community should focus on both women and men, rich and poor, the strongest local institutions which may, depending on the situation, include water and sanitation committees, health services, schools and their children, PRIs, ICDS, savings and youth groups, women clubs and so on. An enabling environment is needed at the intermediate and macro-levels to ensure that new capacities can be practiced. It is not a choice between supporting capacity in the community or block, or district or state level, but for capacity support at all levels (Bossuyt, 1995).

Schouten and Moriarty (2003) have called the intermediate level that support communities' work that 'vast fuzzy region that lies between national/state and local . . . communities' (p. 161). In India, this can include:

- Government: District and block level government apparatus and line departments such as Public Health Engineering, Rural Development, Education, ICDS;
- Institutions: training and teacher training, IEC units, rural development, universities;
- Block officials of the line departments;
- PRIs and personnel;
- NGOs, grassroots organizations, local branches of larger NGOs;
- Private sector: consultants, contractors, service providers;
- Others: CBOs, professional associations, and independent regulators.

Methods: How to support the development of people's capacity? Capacity development includes, but goes beyond classroom learning and training alone. Other methods which appeared in this programme included learning through:

- exchange and study visits;
- mentoring (someone visits and helps);
- consultancies;
- support from people who have successful experience;
- continuing backstopping or follow-up;
- learning by initiating pilots and experimentation at any level (including construction);
- joint planning activities.

SCOPING: AN INNOVATIVE METHODOLOGY

Scoping was a central methodology of this capacity development programme. It represents a transformation of the concept of scoping that originated in public debates over environmental issues in North America. In that context public involvement is used to determine the boundaries of crucial environmental issues, that is, the problem areas, the critical resources and how problems, resources and solutions interrelate.

This scoping strategy was adopted, then adapted and developed by Indian leaders and professionals from eight states and the Government of India, facilitated by UNICEF and IRC/WEDC. The concept was to create the opportunity for representatives of district institutions and groups to think, plan and act together with a focus on removing obstacles to sector reform by using local resources. Scoping is a coordinated planning process that matches obstacles to resources to form a district capacity development plan prepared in a workshop setting by representatives from district institutions/groups and by district leaders. The scoping, described in detail subsequently, is a strong capacity development exercise in itself and results in an action oriented plan. It matches obstacles/gaps with resources and combines training with joint planning.

The result of the scoping activity is more practical and broader in vision than a needs assessment or a training plan. A scoping strategy was selected and adapted, rather than a needs assessment, as the outcome of a training needs assessment, tends to be a long list of activities that is so discouraging that action can hardly be taken. Scoping works to solve the identified challenges through the use of identified, locally available, resources. It is formulated to lead to immediate action for district, block and community capacity development.

INDIAN WATER AND SANITATION SECTORS REFORM

In 1999, the GoI, its Ministry of Rural Development and the Rajiv Gandhi National Drinking Water Mission committed themselves to reforming the rural water supply and sanitation sector.

Water Reform

Despite the high recorded coverage of drinking water facilities achieved in India during previous decades, services had not achieved the expected results in terms of sustainability and health benefits, nor were people fully satisfied. In response to this, reforms were being introduced to move the sector away from a centralized, supply-driven approach towards one that is decentralized, community-oriented and demand-responsive, so that users get the service they want and for which they are willing to pay. Under the reforms, rural water supply systems were to be managed by user groups. Twenty per cent of the annual outlay under India's national Accelerated Rural Water Supply Programme (ARWSP) was earmarked for projects to institutionalize community-based rural water supply systems based on the following principles (RGNDWM, 2000):

- Adoption of a demand-responsive and adaptable approach based on empowerment of villagers to ensure their full participation;
- Shifting role of government from direct service provider to enabler;
- Minimum 10 per cent user contribution to capital costs (in cash or kind or both) and full user responsibility for O&M;
- Broad elements of the reforms included:
  - Preparation of district action plans;
  - Adoption of participatory methods;
  - Capacity development of PRIs and local communities;

- IEC related to hardware and software aspects;
- Monitoring and evaluation; and
- Special attention to water quality, source sustainability.

TOTAL SANITATION CAMPAIGN

The Total Sanitation Campaign (TSC) is a reform of the national rural sanitation programme (Restructured Centrally-sponsored Rural Sanitation Programme). TSC seeks to bring about an improvement in the general quality of life in the rural areas by:

- Accelerating coverage of rural population;
- Stimulating demand through awareness creation and health education;
- Covering schools in rural areas with sanitation facilities;
- Encouraging suitable cost effective and appropriate technologies; and
- IEC to promote sanitation as a means to achieving a better quality of life.

As with water, the programme was planned as community led and people centred, with emphasis on awareness building. A demand-driven approach was adopted with the intention to gradually phase out subsidies for household latrine units. The restructured programme differed from earlier efforts in:

- Offering a broader range of technologies and technology improvisations with reference to customer preferences, construction materials and capacities;
- Developing back-up services such as sanitation production centres (PC), rural sanitary marts (RSM), trained masons;
- Stressing on software, including intensive IEC campaigns in the context of 'total sanitation campaigns';
- dovetailing the range of funds from GoI and state programmes aimed for rural development; and
- fostering broader participation including NGOs, civil society organizations and CBOs (GoI, 2001).

Unlike the water reforms, however, the latrine aspects of the sanitation effort faced fundamental challenges of low levels of coverage (less than 20 per cent) and low demand.

In India, each district has roughly 2 million people, divided into local government areas (blocks and Panchayats) of varying sizes. Seventy-two districts were the focus of the pilot water reform effort. More than 115 districts were designated as 'sanitation districts' with growth to 200 by the end of 2002. This implies that some districts had either water or sanitation reforms, while others had both.

A few states and districts began to implement the water and sanitation reforms in full. Some completed policy frameworks; some started with internal capacity building; others were able to just make a start. Financial resources were sent and a major challenge was the use of funds wisely in the gradual devolution of power to district and Panchayat levels.

Programme Strategy and Activities

In 2001, when this programme for capacity building was developed, the reforms, at the time less than three years old, were seeking to put in place a decentralized framework throughout India to ensure sustainable, safe drinking water supply and effectively-used sanitation facilities with relevant hygiene behaviours. The focus of this programme was capacity building at the relevant levels of responsibility to support and move this extraordinary undertaking forward.

STRATEGY AND START

Within the overall context of reform and decentralization, the capacity building programme was designed with the aim of focussing on building upon existing experience, ensuring capacity is in place and learning how to move to scale while retaining quality. Capacity building plays a pivotal role as without it, efforts for change will gradually be undermined by reversion to old, known institutional behaviour. In 2001, senior personnel from the Rajiv Gandhi National Drinking Water Mission, from UNICEF-India and IRC developed the initial plan, a three-step process (UNICEF and IRC, 2001):

- To organize and plan with a national core team which would serve as the 'motor' for the programme;
- To develop scoping at the district level facilitated by core team members. This was seen as a joint district training-and-planning

process that would develop practical capacity development plans, which would be approved by all representatives of all district stakeholders;
- Dissemination to other districts.

The goal was to attempt to 'jump-start' effective capacity development, first on a pilot level and then to disseminate this.

In the initial meeting, it was decided to address both water and sanitation reforms simultaneously in the capacity development programme. At the district level and in villages, water and sanitation are dealt with by the same groups and similar stakeholders. Furthermore, water and sanitation are intimately connected within the household and at the individual behavioural level. Therefore, these two aspects were addressed simultaneously in the reform process, taking advantage of the synergy between the two.

Based on the decisions taken in this initial meeting, IRC developed a draft concept paper which was then reviewed and revised in detail by both the GoI and by UNICEF, resulting in many improvements. This detailed revision also demonstrated the high degree of ownership by all parties, something which continued throughout the life of the programme. A team of facilitators was then contracted by UNICEF from IRC and WEDC. As these were outsiders, it was agreed that they would work along with the core team as close colleagues, not in the traditional fashion as consultants. UNICEF provided support for the external inputs to the programme, while the GoI supported the district-based activities. Table 9.1 provides an overview of the main elements of this capacity development programme, including who was involved, how that element of the programme was developed and what support products were used.

INITIAL WORKSHOP

Fifteen people were identified by the GoI to attend a two-week Core Team Workshop. The participants were drawn from the government, UNICEF, state training and rural development institutions, state PHED and rural development as well as NGOs. This mix of professionals resulted in a lively and productive workshop. The purpose of the workshop, held in the Netherlands, was to plan the capacity development programme and share experiences among the members

Table 9.1: Main Elements of the Capacity Development Programme

What	Who	How	Support Products
Central motor to support capacity development	Core group, combining public and private membership. People of proven expertise in community management and decentralization.	Forge a group through learning/planning workshop. Frequent review and planning sessions at Centre. Deploy in small teams to districts.	List institutions. Show outline of workshop. Indicate how deployed.
Key objectives of decentralization agreed at all levels.	Leaders in Centre, state leaders, leaders in districts, sub-districts, communities.	Consultation and advocacy at Centre. District meetings with department leaders. One-page summary of reforms, prepared in iterative process.	One-page summary, list of consultation and meetings with comments.
Strategy for capacity development: Key to implementing decentralization.	Representatives of all stakeholders: Panchayat, block officials, training institutions, CBOs (SHG groups, etc.), NGOs, district officials for PHED, education, DRD, ground water.	Scoping: Activity for training with planning scoping works to identify and match local needs with local resources, examine own best experience and institutions, examine needs and problems in WES sector. Field trip is essential. Combine these inputs to make CD plan.	Scoping workshop plan.
Advocacy and policy	District collector, department heads, state leaders.	District leader meetings. State debriefing. National advocacy. Including political leaders.	Packet for district leaders. Note of meetings at state/ national levels.
Management	DSU (district support unit)	In the advocacy and planning process at the district level, stakeholders see that a DSU is needed for decentralization of the sector.	
Follow-up	By institutions of core team members and others.	Training consultancy, membership DSU on demand of district institutions.	

of the core team. These core group activities were also meant to help broker a more productive relationship between NGOs, government, and institutions involved in the sector. Subsequently, however, only about half of the participants were fully active in the programme. Others were transferred, or not in a position to contribute, or were not fully committed to the concept.

THE SCOPING PROCESS

The active members of the core team including IRC/WEDC were split into groups to conduct scoping workshops in the districts. Usually three to five core team members visited each district for a period of seven to eight days. The first workshops were used to design and test the scoping methodologies. In the last scoping workshops, a draft manual was tested. The Indian core team members were the lead facilitators.

District-level scoping was conducted in six districts in all regions of India. It was a participatory learning and planning process aimed at developing a district-specific capacity development plan for the implementation of the water supply and sanitation reforms. Each scoping resulted in capacity development plan for all sectors and levels and included training of the intermediate-level personnel, field visits and repeated consultations/briefings of district leaders.

- The tailored scoping process used in this programme was a dual-faceted activity comprising the scoping activity and the meetings with district leaders detailed above. During the five-to-seven-day scoping workshops, key obstacles operating against sector decentralization as well as specific resources to address identified obstacles were examined. The workshops had between 30 to 70 participants. Table 9.2 gives an example of a workshop programme.

The programme varied somewhat according to local circumstances and experiences in earlier scoping workshops. The scoping activities included the following:

- Background: concepts and introduction to water and sanitation sector reforms;
- Who is involved in water and sanitation reforms: actor analysis;

Table 9.2: Example of a Workshop Programme in a District

Day	Sessions
1	Introduction Understanding sector reform issues and procedures. Explanation of what is scoping and capacity development.
2	Stakeholders' analysis, with future roles under the reforms. A first identification of obstacles to sector reform and resources for capacity development.
3	Field visit to a. communities; b. block-level institutions and resource agencies; c. district-level institutions and resource agencies. The objectives are to validate the stakeholders analysis, to identify constraints with reform implementation; and to identify resources (expertise).
4	Revision of obstacles and resource analysis from day two organized by expected results of the reform. This revision is used to begin making plans that are relevant to different levels (community, block, district, SO).
5	Devising of a capacity development plan by expected results. This plan provides an integrated vision and orientation of what is needed for this district.
6	Review of plan and highlighting priority activities for the coming six months. Closing of workshop.

- Participants identified main obstacles and bottlenecks for sector reform;
- Field trip to collect information and to have a 'reality check' on the scoping work;
- Participants identified 'good' resources: successful examples, useful experience, the people and institutions that can help; and
- Participants made a district capacity development plan that matched the resources with the needs.

BACKGROUND

To start off, the concepts were discussed and the water and sanitation sector reforms were introduced. Information materials about the reform process were simplified and tailored to assist in the capacity building and planning processes. Very simple information is seldom available and few people have access to or read lengthy manuals or policy documents written in complex way. Therefore, a 'one-pager' defining outputs, processes and indicators was very useful

(Table 9.3). It was easily shared and served as a tool to establish common understanding of the issues at hand and agreed objectives for the programme among a large number of people. The one-page overview had been carefully reviewed and edited by leaders of the water and sanitation sectors in the Government.

ACTOR ANALYSIS

The analysis began with brainstorming and then examined the groups identified more carefully. Initially, in some districts it was assumed that the key actors were the water committees, user groups and the PHED. The results of this work usually lead to the following types of conclusions about capacity development and roles in the programme:

- At community level: Capacity development in the community should focus on women and men, rich and poor, the strongest local institutions which may, depending on the situation, include water and sanitation committees, health services, schools and their children, local government (PRI), early childhood care and education (ICDS), savings and youth groups, women clubs and so on. An enabling environment is needed at the intermediate and macro-levels to ensure that new capacities can be practiced. It is not a choice between supporting capacity in the community or block, or district or state level, but for capacity support at all levels (Bossuyt, 1995).
- At intermediate level: The people involved in supporting communities work at the intermediate level are a large group of institutions and individuals lying between the State and community. This can include at the district level:
    - The leaders of district line departments such as public health engineering, rural development, local government, education, early childhood, women and health;
    - The staff of these departments; and
    - Semi-governmental institutions such as universities, mass media institutions, and teacher training colleges.
- At block level: officers from the line departments in the district and local government administrators.

Other intermediate level institutions may be:

- NGOs, grassroots organizations, local branches of larger NGOs;
- Private sector: consultants, contractors, service providers; and
- Others: CBOs, professional associations, and independent regulators.

Table 9.3: Handout Defining Expected Results and Key Indicators of Sector Reform

COMMUNITY LEVEL	
People participate in decision-making	Men and women, rich/poor, members of all communities are all informed, attend meetings, make plans and decisions. Maps or baseline information are easily available, used and understood. Stronger CBOs, formal and informal groups in community are mobilized. Initial contribution for water service from all user groups.
Committees function well	Committees represent all people in the community. Have clear rules, meet, decide and act on own decisions. Community knows what committees do. Committees are linked clearly to the Panchayat and other committees.
Good use and control of money	Payments and collection of funds is rapid and fair for rich and poor. Public display of financial information and programme progress. Payments and collections are accounted and explained to men and women. Has independent financial, physical and social checks/audits.
Water supply functions well	Consistent supply of water (daily, monthly, throughout the year). Technology choice involved men/women. Construction/rehabilitation is low cost and follows standards and norms. Speedy repairs of breakdowns. Maintenance. Rich and poor people make regular payments, enough for capital costs and O&M. They get good service/access to safe water: quantity, water resources (recharge and right to use water), quality of water.
Stronger sanitation demand	Strong demand through intensive IEC promotes high household latrine coverage. Choice of technology options includes low-cost latrines and special conditions (example: high water tables). Construction is good, low-cost with access to hardware (e.g. sanitary marts). Latrines are maintained, clean and used by all family members. No exposed excreta.
Consistent hygiene behaviours	Correct hand washing at critical times by all. Face washing. Bathing. Use and maintenance of latrines. Disposal of child's stools.

	Water hygiene. Use of safe water sources (collection, storage, use of water). Area around water source is clean.
School and Anganwadi programmes	Teachers/parents are informed before construction, support and influence technology/design before construction. Latrines, drinking and hand washing facilities. Latrine design is simple but strong with enough facilities for children. Separate facilities for boys/girls. School children, boys and girls consistently use latrine, hand washing and drinking facilities. Good maintenance with help of children and teachers. Hygiene education in class by trained teachers. Hygiene promotion from schools and children to home.
SUPPORT LEVEL	
Effective IEC, demand creation	IEC combines mass and personal communication with appealing messages (not only health) for different groups. NGOs, government and community groups lead demand creation. Adequate time is given for IEC before construction. Demand for latrines and good use of latrines and water increases.
Local government is responsive	District/Block/NGO knowledge of SR rules and policy and ability to make these known to community members. Transparent community selection, rules known. District and block officials able to respond quickly and clearly to local plans. They are skilled at communicating and know content subjects, technologies, and so on. Timely, transparent, correct release of funds. Correct reporting. Post-construction management support continues in communities.
Effective support organizations	Good facilitation by women and men, including those working at district, block and in NGOs who take part in regular capacity development. Transparent selection and supervision procedures for construction and support contracts. Adequate time frame for project and contracts. Realistic workloads and reporting. Post-construction follow-up: continued supervision and community visits. Help solve problems and have refresher training.

IDENTIFICATION OF MAIN OBSTACLES AND BOTTLENECKS

Obstacles identified by the participants included technical obstacles such as saline water intrusion along the coast; administrative obstacles such as the slow release of funds, non-transparent panchayat accounting on use of funds; substantive obstacles about how to increase demand for household latrines; and, operational obstacles such as how to involve poor people, how to have gender-sensitive programming, how to ensure that construction costs of latrines are known and are kept as low as possible.

FIELD TRIPS

Each workshop included one or two field trips to Panchayats, villages, NGOs, and block offices where water and sanitation reform activities were underway in order to validate the stakeholders' analysis and identify constraints and resources. Gradually, usually after field trips, participants identify capacity needs of the intermediate level, e.g. block- and district-level staff and institutions who themselves must develop better ways of supporting communities.

The participants identified 'good' resources: successful examples, useful experiences, the people and institutions that can help. Locally available resources that could address identified obstacles included local research or training institutions that give good training on a subject; projects or NGOs working in the area that have effective activities for water, community management and/or sanitation; and, individuals who have proven experience in a particular field. These could come from an institution, or from the government or the private sector.

DISTRICT CAPACITY DEVELOPMENT PLAN

The participants then made a district capacity development plan that matched the resources with the needs. The scoping process included district capacity building plans which identified bottlenecks and needs; clearly stated capacity building priorities (who, what, when); identified resources to support capacity building; and, how to go about building capacity, e.g. training, exchange visits, follow-up activities, and plans for pilots and experiments with costs. Some examples are shown in Tables 9.4 to 9.6. Table 9.5 is for the beginning of a sanitation programme in a district that has little past experience. Table 9.6 is an excerpt from a district capacity development plan presenting an innovative idea: the training/management institution for women's savings groups would be deployed to train hamlet water and sanitation groups in bookkeeping and then to check the books, helping ensure transparency and good control of funds. The table's contents will be

Table 9.4: Excerpt from Plan: Objective and Activities for Water Technologies

Objective: Water supply services effective

(1)	(2)	(3)	(4)	
Constraints	Activities	Stakeholders by level	Facilitators and resources	
			From within district	From outside district
Communities are not aware of different technologies with merits, demerits, costs, O&M for source protection, wells, boreholes, etc.	Activity 1 Hamlet meetings to make HWSC and HWSG aware of different technologies with merits, demerits source protection.	HWSG, HWSC	Staff and RW Engineer (by name)	
	Activity 2 Training and planning for technology choices, people-friendly plans, O&M costs.	SO staff and RWS Engineer		ESCI, ASCI APARD can organize CD for SO + RWS

mandatory before the hamlet water and sanitation committee can receive its first instalment. It was decided to divide the awareness creation training separated from skill training. There will also be a pilot to see if these can be combined. The suggested timing to start was as soon as possible.

WOMEN PARTICIPANTS

It was important to have women in the scoping workshops. Their view of water and sanitation tended to differ from that of men, and their jobs as well. Without the active participation of women, some major information and strategic ideas would have been lost. At the start of the workshops, facilitators asked district leaders or district linking officer to ensure that more than four women were present throughout the workshop, from at least three different institutions/ levels (e.g. local government, rural development, Self Help Groups,

Table 9.5: Excerpt from Plan: Sanitation

Objective: To start a strong sanitation demand and programme

(1)	(2)	(3)	(4)	
Constraints	Activities	Stakeholders by level	Facilitators and resources	
			From within district	From outside district
Little is known or done about house-hold latrines and hygiene behaviours such as hand-washing	Study visits within and outside the district	Member Secretary, DWSC members, DSU, NGO-leaders	NGO (name) in district	Midnapore project, West Bengal
	Plan district/block strategy to create demand-driven sanitation programme	DWSC members, DSU, NGO-leaders		
	Training/ orientation	NGOs, PHED, CBOs, schools, blocks,		
	Total Sanitation Campaign, start on small scale	Women, men, households, PRIs	NGOs, PHED, CBOs, schools, blocks	

ICDS). During the opening sessions, facilitators counted the number of women participants and in some cases activities only commenced once the requisite number of women was present as the scoping results would not be representative or reliable without sufficient involvement of women. One strategy used to increase the profile of women's inputs and ideas was to have a man help the women make presentations.

DISSEMINATION

Briefings about the scoping process and outcomes (with advocacy) were held at the state level for leading government personnel; and, at the national level for representatives of a wide range of institutions.

Table 9.6: Bookkeeping and Accountability

Issue	Step	Result	Resource Facilitator	Audience	How	Where	Facilitator Needs	Indicative Cost
Lack of materials	**Step I:** Preparation of materials on detailed book keeping, accounts	District Resource team prepares training materials	Resource Team (10): DSU. NGO (Speak Remede), APO DRDA	–	4-day workshop to collect and prepare training materials from other districts and states	District level	–	10 mandays x 4 = 40 @ 200 = Rs. 8,000 + 2,000 mats TOTAL = Rs. 10,000
Money management and accountability	**Step II:** Training of Trainers (TOT)	Teams of trained and skilled trainers developed	Resource Team (10): DSU. NGO (Speak Remede), APO DRDA	G.P. Secretary; Motivator (92 x 2 = 184) field staff of MACTS 10 Total: 194	2-day classroom with dummy practice. Visit to MACTS.	District Level 5 batches.	–	194 x 2 = 388 + 20 trainers = 408 408 @ Rs. 200 = Total Rs. 81,600
	Step III: Implement-ation	Treasurer and 2 other members of the HWSC, know book keeping and accounting.	G.P. Sec., Motivator, Field staff of MACTS	Nominees from HWSC @ 3 (276 members)	2 days. Little classroom practices. Role play by SHG.	Block level. 5 batches. 2 trainer teams.	–	276 x 2 = 552 + 24 Trnrs = 576 576 @ Rs. 150 = Total Rs. 86,400

Spot checks and community monitoring	**Step IV:** Spot village visits, financial monitoring and refresher training	Books, payments, tenders, receipts; transparent and well managed.	G.P. Sec., Motivator, field staff of MACTS	HWSC and communities.	Spot checks of HWSC: books, payments, receipts with on-site refresher training. Backstopping is needed	Begins after training	Need clear channels for reporting results and taking action.	To be planned.

This was a more limited form of dissemination than had originally been foreseen as the programme ended earlier than planned.

END OF THE PROGRAMME

In mid-November 2002 the national policy regarding water sector reform was changed. This was not foreseen by the people who were working on the scoping activities and capacity development programmes. The new policy appeared to de-emphasize software, capacity development, joint planning, and collaboration among departments on the reform. Members of the core group who had, to a large extent been working in a semi-voluntary way, decided to disband. Thus, the last programme activity, a dissemination 'training of trainers' for scoping in additional districts was not held and thus, this capacity development project was not completed.

One half-year later the national policy was again changed, reverting to lines quite similar to the pre-November 2002 programme. However, by then it was too late to revitalize the capacity development project.

Results and Outputs

The outputs of the programme were disappointing compared with what might have been expected if the capacity development project had been completed. Nonetheless, there were some tangible outputs and results.

First, a strategy was developed and tested to initiate broad, large-scale capacity development at district level, through scoping. It was decided to carry out pilot scoping activities in seven different districts of India (Ganjam in Orissa; Nellore in Andhra Pradesh; Mehsana in Gujarat; Sehore, in Madhya Pradesh; Alwar in Rajasthan; Sirmour in Himachal Pradesh, and Haridwar in Uttaranchal).

Second, there is real evidence that the plans made during the capacity development project are actually being implemented in three of the six districts where the scoping took place. Such plans reflect lessons learned from scoping as in Ganjam, Orissa (Table 9.7). About 300 people received training about sector reform and made plans to implement it in the seven districts. In addition, approximately 60 district and 50 state leaders were oriented (and 'advocated') and they provided important inputs to the programme. Some implementation in half of the areas is what was roughly expected during the development of the new programme. Interestingly, in one district programme, activities were used to develop the institutional arrangement for the sanitation and water sectors, bringing a large project into a working relation with the government programme. The subsequent impact of this capacity development project on the quality of decentralization reforms in the three active districts where the coping plans were implemented.

Third, scoping activities, or similar training-cum-joint planning activities, have reportedly been undertaken in some other districts not involved in the pilot phase. Observers have mentioned six other districts to the authors. In Madhya Pradesh, UNICEF and the government continued scoping in all districts—about 20 out of 46 districts have been completed thus far.

Furthermore, a manual with details on the content and methodology of the scoping programme was completed (Brikké and Shordt, 2002). Also included are information and materials for district leaders as well as details on how to use specific participatory methods in a scoping workshop.

Finally, there were also some unexpected results. For example, the national government and some district governments have asked for continuing services from a small number of the national core teams. Also, some of the professionals involved in scoping at the district level have been promoted to leadership positions in sector reform, in part because of their affiliation with the capacity development programme.

LESSONS LEARNED ABOUT SCOPING

The following is a selection of lessons learned from the UNICEF programme in the state of Orissa, which remain relevant for the overall project.

General Lessons about the Process

One of the strengths of the programme was that it involved many local institutions and groups that have experience and skills to offer. It is not adequate to give the responsibility for support to one group such as government personnel. Involving NGOs and CBOs also

Table 9.7: Six Major Lessons about Scaling Up Community Management in Ganjam, Orissa

1. In community management, decision making, including financial control, should be devolved to the community level.
2. Decision making means that communities have choices. Systems are needed so that people can make informed choices among options.
3. Community management needs quality facilitation. Quality cannot or should not be sacrificed to achieve quantitative targets because, in the long run, this is wasting of resources and leads to failed programmes.
4. Community management requires support, above all, from political leadership. This can help change the top-down attitude of the intermediate level government to service delivery.
5. The capacity of local NGOs to facilitate community processes is great.
6. Scaling up of community management needs partnership with communities, NGOs and the government working to achieve common objectives.

(IRC, 2002, p. 33)

provide a stronger voice for the poor and for women with whom these institutions tend to work. About the methodology, it was found that training needs to be combined with joint planning as it cannot be taken for granted that those responsible for reform implementation know what sector reform or sanitation means.

- Scoping—and support for reforms in general—at the district level should have two focal points. First, commitment of district leaders is built through advocacy and agreeing and the plans being developed. Their support is essential for the success of the programme. Second, focus on those who will carry out and plan the activities, usually mid-level district and block government, NGO staff, CBO personnel and institutional staff. The point is to combine training and advocacy with joint planning.
- Capacity development tools that go beyond training through the use of joint planning, field and exchange visits, consultancies on special issues, and local scoping in blocks are also of great value. The field trip in particular allows participants to see the best of NGO and PHED projects as well as to investigate needs at block and panchayat levels.
- The details and objectives of the process of reform need to be available to those responsible for implementation within the districts, in an appropriate format using simple terminology. At the time of this programme, some districts had water reform

and some had TSC, while others had both. Understanding about the reform process by different stakeholders differed greatly and hampered coordination of planning and implementation. Additionally, objectives of reform (e.g. better service, faster service, use of service, reaching the poor, and reaching areas of low water and/or sanitation coverage) are not generally agreed upon and capacity to implement decentralization is frequently lacking. One effective devise was the simple one-page summary of the key outputs and indicators of sector reform depicted in Table 9.2.

- Involvement of women is essential, particularly those involved in CBOs, health and education sectors and local government. There is a tendency for nearly all participants to be male. Involving women who have relevant experience results in a broader vision and improves the quality of the plans. Sometimes, however, women are not listened to or may have difficulty expressing themselves. Therefore, specific attention and efforts for their involvement and visibility are required.
- The scoping builds a strong sense of ownership in a district or block through collaborative planning and learning. It motivates participants in the group planning process, to think of new ways to address continuing needs and problems; and, to avoid falling back on old ways of doing things that were unsuccessful.
- Finance matters must remain central to the considerations about an enabling environment. This will enhance quality and ensure greater attention to gender and equity aspects of service delivery by local government or other actors. Furthermore, checks and balances are also needed to ensure transparency.
- The quality of the scoping workshops varied. The plans made in the seven districts in part seemed to reflect differences among the districts and facilitators of the scoping activities in each district. Where one department, such as the PHED, had great dominance in the district reform programme, then the scoping workshops and scoping plans were less successful.
- A general rule for similar programmes is to keep the process simple! The scoping activity lasted five to seven days in a district, and involved many participatory activities, joint planning and one or two field trips. However, this is probably too expensive and difficult to organize in most districts. This could limit its

potential for dissemination to other districts. A three, or four-day programme, including a field trip, would be more feasible and practical.

General Lessons about the Enabling Environment

In any setting, the process of decentralization requires consistent policies. In this case, the capacity development efforts ended due to an abrupt change of policy.

- Lessons about motors, management and institutional arrangements in districts:
    - The scoping reports often called for improving district institutional arrangements for sector reform in the district. A 'motor' is needed to keep the sector reform vehicle running. However, if the driving force behind the reform is one individual, and that individual is transferred or retired, then the whole sector reform is in danger. The new person may have other interests or be unfamiliar with sector reform. Therefore, it is better, at the district and block levels, to have a small committed group guiding the reform process.
    - Having an active ZP/DWSM and a DWSC, assisted by a professional core group or District Support Unit is invaluable for facilitating the execution of the water/sanitation reforms, in general, and the capacity development plans, in particular, in a district. Permanent district teams such as the District Support Units are needed to guide and support the process. It is useful to have some dedicated staff that can form a District Support Unit to facilitate the reform. They should be skilled and should carry enough authority to be able to create synergy by ensuring convergence amongst the various line departments in the district.

- Lessons regarding state level

  A similar driving force must exist at the state level. The state-level driving force will be required to closely follow the execution of the capacity development plan in the district, and extend state support and guidance from time to time. Such state institutions can also help the districts link up to different resource institutions in other districts and other parts of the nation.

- Panchayats

  Similarly, at the Panchayat and village level also, there has to be a properly constituted body with due representation of the user groups as well as the PRIs. To ensure an effective reforms process, there should be clear demarcation in the responsibilities and powers of the individuals, and leadership of the institutions leading the reforms.
- Follow-up Support
  - Follow-up is needed, at district, block and panchayat levels. This can serve to monitor the capacity development and its quality, for trouble-shooting and for further development inputs. It is important for an external agency to conduct regular reviews of the process. For instance, a specially constituted review mission comprised of the facilitators who conducted scoping in the district could visit the state, as well as district, to meet the key stakeholders. A meeting with the scopers along with a field visit could also be done to review the impact of the plan in the field.
  - Support from the centre: Senior staff from the Department of Drinking Water (and Sanitation) were, together with UNICEF, committed to the programme. They visited most of the districts during the scoping activities, and some facilitated, with skill, the scoping workshops. This support was invaluable.
- Core Team

  The core group needs to have a mix of public, semi-governmental and private membership and selection of the best practitioners is crucial. In the programme in India, it is important to note that the work of the core group of skilled Indian professionals who led and designed the scoping programme was of highly professional quality and the group deserved official recognition and adequate remuneration. However, the selection process should have been improved to ensure that more of the 15 original participants could have become committed and productive members of this group.

- External Facilitators

  The vision and understanding of the external facilitators contracted to guide the process is important. In this case, developing and piloting of the scoping procedures in the first districts was slowed down due to difficulties in forging a common vision and understanding of the scoping process and ways of working with district participants. Consequently, the process of developing practical plans at the district level for follow-up after the scoping activity took a great deal longer than anticipated.

CONCLUSION

This case study has presented the conceptual underpinnings, implementation experiences and outcomes of a programme to scale up capacity building activities in the context of reform of the water and sanitation sectors in India. The approach taken by this programme is of interest for the emphasis it placed on the building of capacity at the intermediate (district) level of government in order to enable that level to provide improved support to communities that play a significant role in the management and provision of their own water and sanitation services.

The programme is also interesting as the approach to identifying capacity building needs was somewhat unique, applying a scoping technique where stakeholders came together in a workshop to jointly think, plan and act on identifying capacity needs, obstacles and local resources to address these obstacles within districts (and states). The lessons learned may offer insights to others who attempt to mount capacity development programmes in support of large-scale efforts for community-managed water supply and sanitation services.

NOTE

1. The contents of this paper present the opinions and views of the author and not of GOI, UNICEF or those involved in the programme.

REFERENCES

Bossuyt, F., 'Capacity Development: How can Donors Do it Better?', ECDPM Policy Brief No. 5, Maastricht, 1995.

Brikké, Francois and Kathleen Shordt, 'Scoping for Capacity Development: Guidance Manual' (unpublished document), Delft: IRC International Water and Sanitation Centre, 2002.

Government of India, 'Central Rural Sanitation Programme: Total Sanitation Campaign', New Delhi: Ministry of Rural Development, Department of Drinking Water Supply, 2001.

Grindle, M.S., 'Building Capacity in the Public Sector', *Public Administration and Development*, vol. 15, 1995.

IRC, 'From System to Service—Scaling Up Community Management: Report of the Conference, 12–13 December 2001', Delft: International Water and Sanitation Centre, 2002.

Morgan, A. and P. Qualman, 'Institutional and Capacity Development, Result-based Management and Organizational Performance', CIDA Policy Branch, Ottawa, 1996.

Rajiv Gandhi National Drinking Water Mission, 'Guidelines for Implementation of Rural Water Supply Programme', New Delhi: Department of Drinking Water Supply, Ministry of Rural Development, Government of India, 2000.

Schouten, Ton and Patrick Moriarty, *Community Water, Community Management: From System to Service in Rural Areas*, London: ITDG Publishing, 2003.

UNICEF and IRC, 'Proposal Initiating a Capacity Building Programme for Sector Reform in India', New Delhi: UNICEF; Delft: IRC International Water and Sanitation Centre, 6 October 2001.

CHAPTER 10

Public-Private-People Water Partnerships: The Small and Local View from India

A.J. JAMES AND PATRICK MORIARTY

INTRODUCTION

Most analyses of public-private partnerships (PPP) and financing of water supply in urban India focus on large private sector water companies bidding for and obtaining concessions and licensing for water supply services in towns and cities. In rural India, the job of providing water for domestic use is left largely to government departments, which implement schemes without particular focus on the poor. This paper focusses on the poor, the small and the local, and looks at the problems of the urban and rural poor to access adequate and safe domestic water, small-scale independent providers who 'organize' water supply to the rural and urban poor, and local-level measures to address domestic water supply problems, particularly during summers and droughts.

While official documents tend to focus on the vast amounts of money spent so far by government on improving domestic water supplies and the large percentage of rural habitations that have been 'fully covered' by water supply schemes, independent reviews reveal a less than satisfactory situation, especially for the poor, even in states like Kerala and West Bengal that are relatively well endowed with water resources. The poor are paying for water, willingly or otherwise, whether or not they can afford to, and sometimes more than the better off. Yet, there is a proliferation of innovative approaches by the small-scale private sector (such as water vendors in urban areas and private water sellers in rural areas) and by NGO and donor-supported projects, to provide more reliable water supply.

Improving access to adequate and safe domestic water supplies all year round, and meeting the International Development Goals will require governments to go beyond allocating more money and commissioning more piped water schemes, to piloting and scaling up promising approaches, collecting reliable information on the economics of water supply, validating government information and seeking better operational integration between government departments.

PUBLIC PROVISION OF DOMESTIC WATER

The Government of India (GoI) has mandated the Ministry of Rural Development to provide safe drinking water to all rural habitations by 2004 (GoI, 2002). At first sight, the efforts to improve the access of urban and rural Indians to adequate and safe supplies of water for domestic purposes are impressive, especially in the last two decades. Officially, 88 per cent of all the 14,22,264 habitations in India are now 'fully covered', meaning that the inhabitants of these habitations have access to at least one source for 250 persons, supplying 40 litres per capita per day (lpcd) of water of acceptable quality within 1.6 km radius of their habitation (and 100 metres elevation in hilly areas), as well as 30 lpcd for their cattle. The Five Year Plans and the annual plans of central government ministries and state departments document that large amounts of money have been spent for this purpose. Every year, the GoI and the 35 state governments in India spend more than Rs. 3,800 crores (over € 750 million), with the share of the central government being around 45 per cent. But given a population of 1.027 billion, this is less than €1 per head (see Box 10.1).

However, the degree of acknowledgement in these documents of the problems with moving from 85 to 100 per cent coverage of rural habitations, and with providing adequate water to all urban residents, belies the scale and magnitude of these problems. The first paragraph of the Executive Summary of a six-volume report on Water Resources Management in India brought out by the World Bank and the GoI in 1998-9 (World Bank, 1999a) puts the issue in a stark perspective:

> Water is becoming an increasingly scarce resource in India, yet it continues to be used inefficiently on a daily basis in all sectors, while sectoral demands

(such as in drinking water, industry, agriculture and others) are growing rapidly in line with urbanization, population increases, rising incomes and industrial growth. At the same time, poor and disadvantaged groups remain underserved by the heavily subsidized public services, and must bear increased health risks plus additional costs (in terms of time and money) of obtaining potable water supplies. Women and children are disproportionately affected under these conditions due to their greater role in water collecting activities. There is, furthermore, insufficient water available in most basins to address environmental and ecological considerations or ensure adequate supplies for other non-consumptive uses (such as navigation, religious observances and leisure needs). The current policies and sectoral arrangements are no longer adequate to ensure full provision of both non-consumptive and consumptive water needs at reasonable costs and prices, nor to safeguard the provision of useable water into the future. (p. xi)

The government is aware that sustainability of drinking water supplies is threatened by a number of factors (ibid., p. 150) including:

- Fast depletion of groundwater levels, accentuating problems of arsenic and fluorosis;
- Sources going dry due to deforestation, which in turn reduces recharge of aquifers;
- Poor maintenance of existing water supply systems;
- Low level of people's participation in the operation and maintenance of existing water systems;

Box 10.1: Government Funding for Rural Water Supply

Although rural water supply is a state subject, the Central Government has been providing assistance to state governments, recognising the importance of providing safe drinking water in rural habitations. The major source of funding is the Accelerated Rural Water Supply Programme (AWRSP), although there are other avenues including the Sector Reform Project, the Sub-Missions to tackle water quality problems (e.g., arsenic, fluoride, salinity, iron, nitrate, etc.), and the Prime Minister's Gramodaya Yojana (PMGY) which has component funds for rural drinking water. In addition. the central government funds research and development, information education and communication (IEC) activities, documentation and information provision, management information systems and monitoring and evaluation.

Source: www.ddws.nic.in

- Neglect of traditional practices and systems of water management.

In order to address these problems, and to achieve its mandated objective of providing safe drinking water to *all* rural habitations by 2004, the GoI is working on the following (ibid., p. 150):

- Controlling over-extraction of groundwater;
- Funding repairs and rehabilitation of existing water supply systems;
- Emphasizing community participation;
- Providing funds for the Sector Reform Projects;
- Promoting water as a socio-economic good;
- Building stronger links with the watershed development programmes.

The poor state of the infrastructure means more money is being pumped into leaky buckets, putting a burden on official resources, which are forced into crisis management during periods of acute water shortages. Although the government provides water in tankers and trains to affected rural habitations, it will become increasingly expensive and difficult to find this additional water in future.

While there is no gainsaying that the situation is bleak, and there is no doubt that the government has to change its approach with regard to this massive problem, there is a considerable amount of innovation on the ground in urban and rural India in improving the access of the poor to adequate and safe supplies of water for domestic use. These contain the ingredients for a new approach that could help India achieve the Millennium Development Goals.

PROBLEMS WITH PUBLIC WATER PROVISION IN RURAL INDIA

The impressive government statistics of nearly 90 per cent coverage across some 14 million rural habitations in India conceal several deficiencies in the domestic water supply situation that research studies have brought out in recent years:

- Recurrent droughts become a feature in most parts of semi-arid India, where the over-abstraction of groundwater has led to meteorological droughts bringing on groundwater droughts (Batchelor et al., 2000; Ramamohan Rao et al., 2003; Moench et al., 1999).

- Acute short-term scarcities in summer result from dropping water tables and mechanical failures: pipelines bursting, motors burning out (see, for instance, James, 2001 and James et al., 2003).
- In some parts of semi-arid India, the government uses water tankers to provide villages with drinking water during acute summer droughts, and requisitioning of agricultural borewells for drinking purposes has become routine. Groups of better off villagers often buy water from nearby towns, at rates such as Rs. 500 for a 500 litres metal tank full of drinking water.
- Social barriers to access which are an unwritten and unmentioned part of rural reality in India, with government departments and NGOs alike preferring to provide separate water points for lower and higher castes. But discrimination takes place when supply to either breaks down (e.g. Ramamohan Rao et al., 2003; James, 2001; James and Snehalata, 2002).
- Macro estimates can be misleading, in the absence of proper vetting of the data at the ground level, collected by government agencies (e.g. Ramamohan Rao et al., 2003).
- Maintenance costs are outstripping budgets, given the preference of politicians and bureaucrats alike of spending on new schemes. Apart from the prospect of repeating the capital investment every 10 years or so (depending on the lifetime of piped water schemes), inadequate maintenance restricts the utility of installed infrastructure even during their lifetime (e.g. World Bank, 1999b).
- Water quality problems such as fluoride and arsenic are found in several parts of the country, and most affected communities are either not aware of these problems, or unaware of what to do.[1]
- Poor payments of monetary and non-monetary costs for domestic water where, apart from regular water markets (e.g. Shah, 1993), the poor walk long distances and suffer verbal abuse from farmers when they go to agricultural borewells when regular water supplies fail (e.g. James and Snehalata, 2002; James

et al., 2003). Women pay these costs disproportionately since they are involved in the bulk of water collection all over the country.

Thus, there are real problems with domestic water supply provision on the ground, masked by official statistics and by local government perspectives. This is true even in states that are relatively well endowed with water resources, e.g. Kerala and West Bengal, where there are pockets of acute scarcity.

Part of the reason why government statistics tend to underestimate the problem is that habitation surveys, meant to assess the situation on the ground throughout the 14 million habitations of the country are conducted at large intervals of time: the first one was around 1991 and the second was on-going in 2003. The response of the government is to put more money into building large piped water supply schemes and to counter acute scarcities in summers and during droughts with water brought in by tankers from outside the affected region. This is clearly an unsustainable trend.

PROBLEMS WITH PUBLIC PROVISION OF URBAN WATER SUPPLY

Urban water supply has a high media profile, since the last few decades have seen chronic shortages of water, especially in peak summer, in large cities and towns in India. The Ministry of Urban Development is responsible for this issue at the central government level (Box 10.2), while the Water Supply and Sanitation (or Sewerage) Boards of large city corporations take responsibility in the large cities, and the municipalities look after it in smaller towns. On the ministry's official website (www.urbanindia.nic), information on urban water supply is divided under the heads of Urban Development, under which provisions for mega cities are discussed, and Urban Water Supply and Sanitation, which details the provisions for towns and smaller cities.

The government started the Accelerated Urban Water Supply Programme (AUWSP) in 1993–4 to provide 'safe and adequate water supply facilities to the entire population of towns having population less than 20,000 (as per the 1991 census)'. There are currently 2,151 such small towns in the entire country. Each state government con-

Box 10.2: Urban Water Supply for Smaller Towns and Cities

The central government selects towns and allocates money to different state governments based on criteria that include the population of these towns and the incidence of poverty in the state. Priority is given to towns with:

- a very low per capita supply of potable water;
- very distant or deep water sources;
- locations in drought-prone areas;
- excess salinity, fluoride, iron and arsenic content in the water sources;
- a high incidence of water borne diseases.

Source: www.urbanindia.nic

tributes 50 per cent of the cost for specific piped water schemes, while the Central Government puts in the remaining 50 per cent.

Large cities such as New Delhi, Mumbai, Chennai, Kolkata, Hyderabad and Bangalore have specially allotted funds through the centrally sponsored scheme for infrastructural development in mega cities, which include water supply and sewerage, roads and bridges, city transport and solid waste management. However, water supply which comes under the Department of Urban Development is 'subject to the overall national perspective of water planning and coordination assigned to the Ministry of Water Resources' (GoI, 2003: Point 24).

Despite investments by the GoI and several donor-assisted programmes to improve water supply in towns and cities (totalling over €1.5 billion since 1990) there has been a constant rise in water demand, fuelled by population growth, which has pushed cities to look for various measures to augment drinking water supplies. Every summer, the water problem in urban areas is highlighted in the media. While cities like Chennai, Anantapur, Bellary and Kurnool are known urban hotspots for water shortages in summer, more cities and smaller towns are reporting water scarcity.

Like the situation in rural areas, finding more water for urban users is becoming increasingly expensive, and difficult, but unlike the rural situation there is little acknowledgement by policy makers that there are problems on the ground. The sources of these problems vary as follows:

- *Poor rainfall and hence inadequate inflow to supply reservoirs*: In Chennai, for instance, poor monsoons that do not fill major supply reservoirs such as Chembarambakkan and Red Hills, affect the summer scarcity.
- *Inefficient supply networks*: Badly maintained and old infrastructure results in leaking pipelines and water points. Along with water theft through unauthorized connections, these are the two main sources for unaccounted for water (UFW) losses. While water systems in most developed countries have UFW losses of around 15 per cent, actual losses are much higher in Indian cities. In Bangalore city, for instance, studies put UFW losses at around 40 per cent, with about half this amount being attributed to leakage and half to unauthorized connections (TARU, 1999). In the absence of good data, the attribution of reasons for these losses is almost pure guesswork.
- *Water quality problems:* While old pipelines and poor maintenance also contribute to water quality problems, intermittent piped water supply encourages microbial contamination. None of India's cities have 24-hour piped water supply (TARU, 1999).
- *Scarcity despite plentiful supply in urban slums*: A curious phenomenon observed in Bangalore city was the plentiful supply of public water points (or 'water fountains'), with water often gushing along the gutters and narrow streets. However, discussions with slum dwellers revealed that these did not have potable water and they had to walk to specific water points, often far away from their houses, to collect potable water (James, 2001).
- *Lack of recognition that the poor pay for water*: Studies from all over urban India have documented that the poor pay for water, often more than the better off, though not necessarily only in terms of money. Walking distances to collect drinking water, waiting in queues at water points for supply to start, even at unearthly times (e.g. 2 a.m. in the morning), suffering conflicts with others trying to get water can be calculated as costs in terms of convenience, effort and time (WSP, 1999a). Some poor households in urban slums buy water three days a week at Rs. 8 per bucket (James, 2001).

Part of the problem of poor maintenance and inadequate supplies is insufficient funds. In most cities, water rates are low and collections are notoriously poor. But raising water tariffs is politically unpopular, and in any case affects only legally connected users, and leaves the illegal connections unaccounted for. Municipalities and town Panchayats, the urban local bodies responsible for water supply in smaller towns, are strapped for cash, infrastructure and staff, and often do not have funds to carry out anything other than emergency repairs and maintenance work (Thimmaiah, 2000; Gnaneshwar, 2000; Sarma, 2000; Singh, 2000).

There is recent evidence that water supply may not be an economically viable activity for urban local bodies. This was emphasized at a recent presentation of the World Bank-funded Tamil Nadu Urban Development Project (TNUDP) in New Delhi. This implies that other sources of municipal revenues have to be found to cross-subsidize the provision of water and sanitation in urban areas.

Fuelled by burgeoning and largely unchecked urban demand for water, India's mega cities are looking further and further away for water sources. Bangalore Corporation has initiated several schemes for taking more water from the Cauvery River flowing relatively nearby, while Chennai has a large and expensive scheme to take water from the far away Krishna River in Andhra Pradesh, and Hyderabad wants water from the Godavari River several hundred kilometres to its north. New Delhi, on the other hand, is pushed to drilling more and more borewells since it cannot take more water from the Yamuna River. What is often overlooked, perhaps wilfully, given the political significance of the urban vote bank, is that these rivers are the sources for the piped water supply to several smaller towns and villages en route, and thus, expansion of mega city water demand may be at the cost of other, perhaps less politically significant urban and rural populations. In Anantapur district in Andhra Pradesh, for example, a piped water supply scheme designed to provide water to Uravakonda, a small town, and five nearby villages could no longer provide water to the villages since the urban demand from Uravakonda had risen sharply in recent years. Such rising demand for urban water is clearly unsustainable.

PARTNERSHIPS TO FINANCE DOMESTIC WATER SUPPLIES

Till recently, the GoI insisted on providing domestic water without charge, as it felt that access to potable water was a basic right. As noted above, however, several studies have documented payments for domestic water in rural India, and have noted that even the poor pay, whether in terms of money or time, effort and convenience.

Supplementary arrangements for domestic water supply operate in several parts of rural India, ranging from private water vendors to community-run multi-village water schemes. Moreover, with the government opening the doors to community-managed water supply schemes through the recently launched Swajaldhara scheme, there are more possibilities for partnerships to finance rural domestic water supply involving government programmes, private providers and rural communities. While no classic PPPs, these are nonetheless significant because they are alternatives to the pure public provision arrangements of the past. And there is evidence to show that rural communities are willing to pay for better water supplies.

The rural poor pay for water in non-monetary ways (e.g. by walking long distances every summer) or with money (e.g. buying water from private water vendors). Today, even government programmes ask rural beneficiaries of piped domestic water schemes to pay 10–30 per cent of capital costs and 100 per cent of maintenance cost. This is the case, for instance, with the Sector Reform Project initiated by the Rajiv Gandhi National Drinking Water Mission of the GoI and carried out in 64 districts of the country from 1999-2002, and scaled up nation-wide in December 2002 as the Swajaldhara drinking water scheme.

Two contingent valuation studies of willingness to pay (WTP) for improved water supplies in rural Gujarat have shown that rural communities are willing to pay for improved water supplies (James and Purushothaman, 1997). But whether or not this would be sufficient to pay for the piped water scheme in the area is not clear. In the WTP study done for the Water Resource Development and Management (WARDEMA) project (James and Purushothaman, 1997), the cost of supply was not fully worked out. Although a review mission from the Royal Netherlands Embassy visited the project after the first phase (1995-8) and recommended the second phase (1999-2003), the project was abruptly cancelled following the Pokharan nuclear test conducted by India in May 1998. There was, thus, no opportunity to complete the detailed technical planning that was required to generate supply cost estimates. In the case of the Gogha Water Supply Project supported by the Royal Netherlands Embassy, total WTP was lower than anticipated cost.

Private providers in urban areas range from tanker suppliers to smaller vendors and even the poor are paying for water, sometimes more than their better-off counterparts, and also in terms of effort, time and convenience. But they are still willing to pay for improved water supply, depending upon the acuteness of the problem and the feasibility of alternative arrangements.

A contingent valuation study of WTP of urban dwellers in Bangalore city (James, 2001) showed that residents were not willing to pay much more than the current water bill of Rs. 100 per month, on average, for a marginally improved supply (three hours everyday instead of only alternate days, convenient hours of supply at guaranteed times instead of varied).

In general, there is pessimism about whether WTP would be higher than 5 per cent of total annual household income, at which level, it may be insufficient on average to costs of supply (World Bank, 1999b).

PUBLIC-PRIVATE-PEOPLE PARTNERSHIPS IN PRACTICE

RURAL AREAS

Alternative arrangements for domestic water supply operate in rural India, involving government programmes, private providers and rural communities. While they are not the classic PPPs, they are nonetheless significant because they are alternatives to the pure public provision arrangements of the past.

Private water societies: In Ollavanna, a village in north Kerala, several groups of households have come together to form private water cooperatives, registered as societies, which supply water to members on payment of a fixed initial contribution and regular monthly collections. However, these are not necessarily poor households.

Community arrangements: In the summer of 2001, the gram panchayat of Inchigeri village in Bijapur district, Karnataka state, arranged to purchase water from a private agricultural borewell after paying the owner Rs. 10,000 (James et al., 2003). In Battuvanipalli village in Anantapur district, Andhra Pradesh state, the gram panchayat negotiated in July 2003 to exchange their high-fluoride drinking water borewell with a farmer's low fluoride borewell, and the payment details are being worked currently. The arrangement was part of the pilot activity of the Water Households and Rural Livelihood (WHiRL) project, a Knowledge-and-Research (KAR) project coordinated by the Natural Resources Institute, UK, and funded by the Department of International Development of the Government of UK.

Community management: Villagers have been running a four-village piped water scheme in Kolhapur district in southern Maharashtra since 1979, when the scheme was completed by the government and handed over to a committee (*mandal*) of villagers (WSP, 1999c). Although the state government department that constructed the system initially was to hand over control to the district government, the district government refused, as no funds had been allocated for the maintenance of the scheme. The junior engineer then went around to the four beneficiary villages, asking them to form a committee (*mandal*) and take over the scheme. To their credit, they did so, and 20 years later they had a profit of Rs. 3 lakhs in the committee bank account. However, a similar 14-village scheme started by the government in a neighbouring set of villages did not do well since the committee failed to pay electricity bills on time, despite collecting money from the villagers. When the state electricity board cut off electricity supply to the village, they took to the streets in protest and brought political pressure to bear on the electricity board officials to get the electricity supply restored. The main reason for the poor performance was that the committee suffered from corruption and mismanagement.

Swayam Shikshan Prayog, an NGO in Maharashtra that also works on community-managed water supply schemes in Latur and Osmanabad districts, reports the following experience in Pardi village: Following a decision by the gram sabha to implement the community participation-based rural water supply and sanitation pilot project, a 12-member Village Water and Sanitation Committee (VWSC) was formed with 50 per cent women participation. Following intensive motivation, mobilization and capacity building, the pilot project involved women members of the gram panchayat, the VWSC, Savings and Credit Groups and *mahila mandals* (women's groups), who actively participated in preparing the scheme, implementation, collecting contributions, maintaining records of the project implementation expenses and monitoring construction work. Such participation from women, who had been largely confined to their own houses prior to the pilot project, has contributed substantially to their own self-esteem and to the possibilities of PPPs in domestic water supply.

To procure pipes for their village water supply system, the chairperson of the VWSC in Kamtoli village in Pithoragarh district in Uttaranchal, a dynamic woman called Shanti Maluda decided to travel 350 km from the hills of Pithoragarh to the Jindal Pipe Factory on the outskirts of Delhi. Shanti Maluda and fellow committee members visited the factory, scrutinized and weighed all the pipes, and took the goods back by truck. Similarly, the committee checked every single fitting and tap, and insisted on replacing any item found without the Indian Standards Institute (ISI) mark (WSP, 2001, p. 4).

Community restriction: In addition to partnerships between local government, farmers and community groups for financing water supplies, there are also instances where the local villagers have persuaded local governments (gram panchayats) to initiate action to protect their drinking water sources. Often these are initiated by NGOs, and in some cases, extended across all villages covered by donor-assisted projects. In several pockets of semi-arid India, gram panchayats have passed resolutions to stop irrigated summer cultivation and to limit the depth of tube wells. Although there are hardly any documented and published cases, NGOs have reported or facilitated such arrangements in several places:

- AFARM (Action for Agricultural Renewal in Maharashtra), an NGO based in Pune, Maharashtra, has been working with villagers to pass panchayat resolutions banning irrigated cultivation in summer, so as to conserve drinking water for acute summer.
- The project video for the WHiRL project has shots of villagers from southern Maharashtra talking about their successes with water harvesting.
- SEWA (Self Employed Women's Association), an NGO in Ahmedabad, mentions that they have helped women in villages in Mehsana district of Gujarat agitate successfully for Panchayat

resolutions banning summer irrigated cultivation and bore wells beyond a certain depth in their villages.

- WOTR in Ahmednagar, Maharashtra, the official Capacity Building and Support Agency of the Indo-German Watershed Development Programme, has made restrictions on bore well depth a precondition for a village being selected for the four-year government-subsidized watershed development programme (www.wotr.org, downloaded December 2003).

Urban Areas

The most common partnership in urban areas is private water vendors, who now operate in several Indian towns and cities. These, however, range from the small pushcart sellers who appear in summer, especially in cities like Delhi, or more regularly in slums in Chennai and Bangalore, to the large water tankers operated by medium-sized private water companies, who buy water from either government sources or private borewells and sell them to individuals by the bucket or as entire tanker loads to restaurants, hospitals and other institutions. Again all these are not the classic PPPs, but have come up to supplement inadequate public provision arrangements.

Private water vendors: Small vendors carry and sell water on bicycles or pushcarts in urban slums, along streets too narrow for larger tankers to traverse. Often they form a distribution system with the main supply being the larger tanker or a public water source of acceptable drinking water quality. Rates charged by these vendors depend on the scarcity of potable water in the locality and can be as high as Rs. 8 per bucket as in Bangalore slums (James, 2001).

Private water tankers: In Chennai and Bangalore cities, the governments use water tankers to provide water to urban residents through the year. While these are free, there are also private water vendors who bring in water from peri-urban areas and charge for their services (WSP, 1998). In recent years, there have been increasing reports of conflicts between these private water companies and villagers from whose lands the water is taken. The Palar River Basin used to supply water to Chennai city is one case in point. However, some villages along the coast of Chennai, from Neelankarai to Sholinganallur, en route to Mahabalipuram, decided to first allow these private tankers, but when they saw the consequences in the form of seawater ingress, they called a halt and cancelled the Panchayat permission they had earlier granted.

Public water tankers: Urban slum dwellers in Bangalore city were WTP 25 paise per litre for tanker-supply with slot machine (like milk booths), stationed outside their slum 24 hours a day and replaced as often as necessary), as opposed to either walking far to collect from potable water points or buying water at Rs. 8 per bucket every alternate day (James, 2001). Men and women in these slums appreciated this idea highly since it meant that they could get water any time they wished, instead of at either fixed but inconvenient timings (e.g. if they left home for work at 7 in and returned at 6 p.m. and water came from 8 to 9 a.m. and 6 to 8 p.m.) or at variable hours. Even if they had to pay for water under the innovative system proposed, they also valued the fact that they would no longer have to request neighbours to collect water for them. This would have paid for the cost of production and distribution of this water, but while the Bangalore Water Supply and Sewerage Board placed this proposal before the cabinet of the State Government of Karnataka, it has not been implemented till date.

Shared taps: Another innovation tried out in Bangalore slums is the shared tap connection, where several households share a single yard tap. All households share the monthly bill equally, although the owner of the yard has the responsibility for paying the bill. Introduced as part of a pilot project, this has apparently been taken up by the Bangalore Water Supply and Sewerage Board subsequently for large-scale implementation (personal communication, Rupa Mukerji, Social Development Unit, Project Management Unit, Bangalore Water Supply and Environmental Sanitation Master Plan Project, Bangalore, October 2002).

Private provision: Although this is not an example from India, the South African experience with the Bambanzi Water Card System appears to be a viable system for regulating water demand, given the experience of the Kamhlushwa township in Malelane district in Limpopo Province. The system consists of a 'water card', which can be bought at the local office and on which payment is 'loaded' as credit, and water meters fitted to public and private taps (e.g. to the main line). Once inserted into the slot in the meter, water flows out of the tap till the card is pulled out (for public taps) or the tap is turned off (for private taps). The meter displays the amount of credit remaining on the card. Additional payment at the local office will result in the card being recharged for further use. Poor women who were using this system in Kamhlushwa stated that it was better than their earlier system of free, but undependable supply, because they no longer needed to go and request neighbours for water, and suffer the indignity of possible refusal. As in the case of slum dwellers in Bangalore, these women prized the opportunity of getting water on their own terms, even if it meant paying for it. The system, however, has not performed well in other parts of South Africa, largely because of inadequate communication and poor handling of popular protests (e.g. Box N in Schouten and Moriarty, 2003).

CONCLUSION: WAYS FORWARD

There is an urgent need to build on the innovative approaches being practiced in different parts of the country. Nearly five years ago, the World Bank—GoI study underscored the need for urgent action. The situation, if anything, is more serious today. Some key ways forward are suggested below:

- *A meta-study to document innovative approaches* to financing domestic water supply in different states of the country. There are several NGO-led approaches and donor-supported projects that are experimenting with innovative schemes for sustainable community-managed water supply systems. Some state and district governments have also been introducing innovative financing and cost recovery systems, but these are poorly documented, inadequately analysed and hardly ever incorporated into new plans and policies being formulated.
- *Reliable economics of water supply* since there is some evidence that rural and urban water supply schemes may not be economically and financially sustainable (i.e. with current costs

including depreciation for future replacement) and hence will require repeated investment to maintain the flow of services. Good quality studies are required to provide reliable answers to the following questions:

- What is the cost of production of water? At what scale?
- What is the extent of subsidy involved?
- What are the 'real' O&M costs with replacement?
- *Validation of official statistics by ground-truthing* since there is evidence (including the Water Resources Audit of the APRLP, Ramamohan Rao et al., 2003) to suggest that official statistics may not be accurate and hence not portraying a correct perspective of ground reality. This is especially important to measure India's progress towards attaining the Millennium Development Goals.
- *Institutional integration exercises* to map the interconnections between the different ministries and departments looking after different aspects of water, to identify institutional and practical bottlenecks and constraints towards an integrated water resource management framework, and to suggest concrete steps and changes in specific policy documents/rules/guidelines to eliminate inconsistencies and contradictions and for better synergy (along the lines of the recent exercise by the European Union to integrating different directives).
- *Piloting of the Bambanzi water meter system in selected urban localities* to work out the optimal mix of capacity building, awareness generation and institutional and financial frameworks required for the effective implementation of this system.

NOTE

1. In the case of arsenic in groundwater, one problem area in India is West Bengal, though it spills over into neighbouring Bangladesh as well. See, for instance, the three field notes on 'Arsenic in West Bengal' brought out by the Water and Sanitation Program (WSP, 2000, 2002a & 2002b) and the recent article in the *Jalvaani* (WSP, 2002c), a newsletter on rural water and sanitation in India, brought out by WSP-SA. A thorough analysis of the fluoride problem in Anantapur district in south India has been carried out by the Water, Households and Rural Livelihoods (WHiRL) Project, details of which are available at www.nri.org/whirl

REFERENCES

Batchelor, C.H., M.S. Ramamohan Rao and A.J. James, 'Karnataka Watershed Development Project Water Resources Audit', KAWAD Report 17, Department for International Development, Government of the UK, and the KAWAD Society, 2000.

Gnaneshwar, V., 'Municipal Functions—The Post-Constitution 74th Amendment Scenario in Andhra Pradesh and Tamil Nadu', *Nagarlok*, vol. XXXII, no. 4, October-December, Special number on Devolution of Functional and Financial Powers to Urban Local Bodies, New Delhi: Centre for Urban Studies, The Indian Institute of Public Administration, 2000.

GoI, *Annual Report 2001-2002*, New Delhi: Ministry of Rural Development, Government of India, 2002, www.ddws.nic.in

———, Task List, Point 24, New Delhi: Department of Urban Development, 2003, www.urbanindia.nic.in/mud-final-site/ministry/index.html

Gopalan, Prema, Director, SSP. Personal Communication, September 2003.

James, A.J., 'Report of the Willingness to Pay Study of Households in Bangalore City for Improved Water Supply and Environmental Sanitation', submitted to TARU Leading Edge, New Delhi, 2001.

James, A.J. and Seema Purushothaman, 'Water Resources Economics and Planning Study', report submitted to the Water Resource Development and Management (WARDEMA) Project in Gujarat, funded by the Royal Netherlands Embassy, New Delhi, 1997.

James, A.J. and M. Snehalata, 'Quantified Participatory Assessments for the Water Resources Audit of the Andhra Pradesh Rural Livelihoods Project', report submitted to DFID India, July 2002.

James, A.J. et al., 'An Integrated Approach to Improving and Protecting Rural Water Supplies in Semi-arid India', paper presented at the National Seminar on Water organized by the Centre for Economic and Social Sciences and the Indian Council of Social Science Research, 30–31 July 2003, Hyderabad, Andhra Pradesh.

Moench, M., Elisabeth Caspari and Ajaya Dixit (eds.), *Rethinking the Mosaic: Investigations into Local Water Management*, Nepal Water Conservation Foundation, Kathmandu, and Institute for Social and Environmental Transition, Boulder, Colorado, 1999.

Nanavaty, Reema, General Secretary of SEWA, Personal Communication, February, 2000.

Ramamohan Rao, M.S. et al. (eds.), 'Andhra Pradesh Rural Livelihoods Programme Water Resources Audit: Phase I Report', Andhra Pradesh Rural Livelihoods Programme and Department for International Development, Government of the UK, 2003.

Sarma, K.S.R.N., 'The Seventy-fourth Constitution Amendment and Municipal Financial Autonomy', *Nagarlok*, vol. XXXII, no. 4, October-December, special number on Devolution of Functional and Financial Powers to Urban Local Bodies, New Delhi: Centre for Urban Studies, The Indian Institute of Public Administration, 2000.

Schouten, Ton and Patrick Moriarty, *Community Water, Community Management: From System to Service in Rural Areas*, London: ITDG Publishing, 2003.

Shah, Tushaar, *Groundwater Markets and Irrigation Development: Political Economy and Practical Policy*, Mumbai: Oxford University Press, 1993.

Singh, U.B., 'Devolution of Functional and Financial Powers to Urban Local Bodies in Uttar Pradesh—A Farce', in *Nagarlok*, vol. XXXII, no. 4, October–December, special number on Devolution of Functional and Financial Powers to Urban Local Bodies, New Delhi: Centre for Urban Studies, The Indian Institute of Public Administration, 2000.

TARU, 'Draft Inception Report, Bangalore Water Supply and Environmental Sanitation Master Plan Project', New Delhi: TARU Leading Edge, 1999.

Thimmaiah, G., Managing the Functions and Finances of Urban Local Bodies', in *Nagarlok*, vol. XXXII, no. 4, October–December, special number on Devolution of Functional and Financial Powers to Urban Local Bodies, New Delhi: Centre for Urban Studies, The Indian Institute of Public Administration, 2000.

World Bank, *Initiating and Sustaining Water Sector Reforms: A Synthesis*, World Bank South Asia Region Rural Development Sector Unit in collaboration with the Government of India, Ministry of Water Resources (Central Water Commission and Central Ground Water Board), Ministry of Urban Areas and Employment, Ministry of Rural Areas and Employment (The Rajiv Gandhi National Drinking Water Mission), New Delhi: Allied Publishers, 1999a.

———, *Rural Water Supply and Sanitation*, World Bank South Asia Region Rural Development Sector Unit in collaboration with the Government of India, Ministry of Rural Areas and Employment (the Rajiv Gandhi National Drinking Water Mission), DANIDA (Danish International Development Assistance), New Delhi: Allied Publishers, 1999b.

WSP, Private Urban Water Suppliers, Field Note, Water & Sanitation Programme—South Asia, New Delhi, 1998.

———, 'Water for India's Poor: Who Pays the Price for Broken Promises?', Water and Sanitation Programme—South Asia, New Delhi, 1999a.

———, 'Villagers Treat Water as an Economic Good', Olavanna, Kerala, India, Field Note, Water and Sanitation Programme—South Asia, New Delhi, SPI Series 4, December 1999b.

———, 'Sustainable Community Management of a Multi-village Water Supply Scheme in Kolhapur, Maharashtra, India, Field Note, Water and Sanitation Programme—South Asia (WSP-SA), New Delhi, SPI Series 2, December 1999c.

———, The West Bengal Pilot Project: Responding to Community Demands for Arsenic-free Drinking Water, Report, Water and Sanitation Programme—South Asia, New Delhi, April 2000.

———, Community Contracting in Rural Water and Sanitation: The Swajal Project, Uttar Pradesh, India, Field Note, Water and Sanitation Programme—South Asia, New Delhi, 2001.

———, Fighting Arsenic, Listening to Rural Communities, Field Note, Water and Sanitation Programme—South Asia, New Delhi, December 2002a.

———, Willingness to Pay for Arsenic-free Safe Drinking Water in Rural Bangladesh—Methodology and Result, Field Note, Water and Sanitation Programme—South Asia, New Delhi, December 2002b.

———, *Jalvaani*, a newsletter on rural water and sanitation in India, vol. 5, no. 3, November 2002-February 2003, Water and Sanitation Programme—South Asia, New Delhi, 2002c.

CHAPTER 11

Sustainable Urban Services and Private Sector Participation: An Indian Experience

V. SATYANARAYANA

INTRODUCTION

The urban sector is poised for major changes through its potential for contributing to India's economic growth. Access to urban water is an important component in urban sector development. Over the last decade, there have been efforts to improve the service and there is recognition of major roles for the private sector and for local communities. However, despite several committed efforts to attract private sector participation, success has been elusive. This paper outlines the past and on-going efforts in sector reforms in general and at attracting private sector participation in particular, and discusses the key considerations in moving this agenda forward.

SERVICE LEVELS OF DRINKING WATER SUPPLY AND SANITATION IN URBAN INDIA

India's population as of 2001 was 1.027 billion with an urban population of 285.35 million. India's urban population forms part of the second largest urban system in the world, next only to China. As per the census of 2001, the service levels in urban areas continue to fall short of the levels that the population desires. Information on service levels for urban water supply and wastewater removal is presented in Table 11.1. Only 50 per cent of the population in urban areas had water taps within the premises. Approximately 65 per cent of households had some sort of water facility, either a tap or well or hand pump, within the premises. The remaining 35 per cent of the population depended on outside sources. On the sanitation front,

61 per cent of households have access to either pit latrines or water closets. Table 11.2 shows that one-quarter of the population did not have access to any sanitation facility. Only 35 per cent of households in cities had access to closed drainage facilities.

Table 11.1: Distribution of Households by Source of Drinking Water and Its Location in Urban India

(in percentages)

Sources of drinking water	Within premises	Near premises	Away from premises	Total
Tap	49.68	15.07	3.91	68.66
Hand pump	8.26	5.89	2.09	16.24
Tube well	2.90	1.36	0.86	5.11
Well	4.36	2.04	1.31	7.71
Tank, pond, lake	0.07	0.12	0.13	0.31
River and canal	0.00	0.10	0.10	0.19
Spring	0.00	0.14	0.11	0.25
Any other	0.12	0.53	0.88	1.52
Total	65.38	25.24	9.38	100.00

Note: Near premises indicates a drinking water source within 100 metres from the premises; away from premises means that the source is located beyond 100 metres.
Source: Computed from GoI (2003).

Table 11.2: Percentage of Urban Households and Availability of Bathroom, Type of Latrine and Type of Wastewater Drainage

Type of service	% households
Households with a bathroom within the house	70.40
Type of latrine within the house:	
Pit latrine	14.60
Water closet	46.12
Other latrine	13.00
No latrine	26.28
Total	100.00
Type of drainage for waste water:	
Closed drainage	34.50
Open drainage	43.37
No drainage	22.13
Total	100.00

Note: 'Other Latrines' include service latrines (which are dry latrines from which human waste is removed by scavengers).
Source: Computed from GoI (2003).

URBAN INFRASTRUCTURE FINANCING

The urban sector in India is the responsibility of the state governments. Traditionally, urban environmental infrastructure such as water, sanitation and sewerage have been considered public services, to be provided by local governments and related parastatal agencies. Therefore, financing of infrastructure has largely been through budgetary allocations, resulting in a lack of rigour in the sector. This has limited the investments, leading to large shortfalls (Mehta and Satyanarayana, 1999).

In the past, municipal authorities have largely depended on grants and loans through budgetary allocations of state and central governments and to a limited extent on surpluses from their own budgets. It is estimated that during the Ninth Plan period (1996–2000), over two-thirds of the financial resources for urban infrastructure came from budgetary allocations. In earlier years, almost the entire financing was through this mode. Institutional finance for these investments is very recent, limited in volume and has been largely through government-owned finance institutions. The local entities, who are the actual service providers, have mostly lacked direct access to the market and any other form of private or institutional finance.

The financing arrangements in India, until recently, have been characterized by a direct credit regime in which different financial institutions are mandated to invest in specific 'priority' sectors (Devi and Satyanarayana, 2002). The government-owned finance institutions (FI) have largely benefitted from this regime, although with the financial sector reforms undertaken during the 1990s this system is now undergoing considerable changes. Resource mobilization by these FIs is being increasingly done through 'market borrowing' without government guarantees. In the urban sector, however, this has been true to a limited extent only for the Housing and Urban Development Corporation (HUDCO). The other intermediaries at the state level have largely depended on state transfers, plan allocations or borrowing from HUDCO for their resources.

Most of the funding has, therefore, come from plan allocations through central and state schemes. Some state governments have provided loans and grants for water supply to local bodies from the allocations. These financing arrangements have resulted in a lack of rigour for lending in this sector. At the borrower's end, this has led to a situation of inappropriate incentives, inefficient utilization of funds and widespread service inefficiencies. There is also a lack of project development and management capacity at the local level. It is common practice that intergovernmental loans are not serviced properly. Such delinquency is often 'solved' by local transfers by the state or the rescheduling of state loans. This has led to a lack of transparency, promoted apathy on the part of the local authorities to financial viability issues, and has meant that inadequate attention is given to effective tariff structures and cost recovery (Mehta and Satyanarayana, 1999).

INVESTMENT REQUIREMENTS AND POTENTIAL

Within the above system, the flow of resources for urban infrastructure has been far too small compared to the requirements. During the Ninth Plan period, the estimated resource flow to the urban infrastructure sector has been only Rs. 50 billion (USD 1.1 billion) per annum with an estimated one-third share of institutional finance. Even these limited funds have not been utilized fully, utilization levels being only 80 per cent. This hints at other constraints in the system, which limit the absorption capacity as well as the low priority accorded to this sector. The institutional capacity constraints do not only limit the absorption of funds, but also result in poor use of funds with inappropriate investments and inadequate planning and project management.

Compared to the likely resource flows, the estimated investments needed in the coming years to upgrade urban infrastructure, including water and sewerage services and roads, is about Rs. 271 billion (US $5.75 billion) per annum at 2001–2 prices over the Tenth Plan period (2002–7). Even after accounting for a trend-based increase in plan allocations and institutional finance, there will be significant shortfalls in relation to the total estimated investment requirements.

Interestingly, however, the resources will be significantly enhanced, if it becomes possible to tap the capital or financial markets. However, to make this a reality will require considerable strengthening of the local institutions as well as major changes in macro-financing arrangements. A number of existing domestic financial institutions, such as ICICI, Housing Development Finance Corporation (HDFC) and the new Infrastructure Development Finance Company (IDFC) have begun to show a keen interest in the urban sector. However, sustaining this will require development of bankable investment opportunities. A major focus in these efforts will have to be on evolving a commercial orientation in urban infrastructure projects and in urban sector institutions.

COMMERCIAL VIABILITY IN URBAN INFRASTRUCTURE SECTOR PROJECTS

The first important aspect, which requires attention to attract investments from commercial investors or lenders to enhance resources for urban infrastructure, is the development of projects in commercial formats. The working definition of commercial viability within the urban sector has evolved over time, based on practical experience in the development of 'commercially viable' projects and a growing understanding of the potential of urban and infrastructure finance sectors. Since 1996, the Indo-USAID Financial Institutions Reform and Expansion (FIRE) Project has strived to work on these aspects. Significant progress has been made in the transition toward a commercial orientation and the demonstration projects developed with assistance from the FIRE Project have succeeded in attracting a substantial portion of their financing from the commercial financing institutions or through direct borrowing from the domestic capital market.

Commercial Financing Arrangements

A variety of project financing arrangements has been developed under the FIRE Project, which ensure commercial viability and bankability of investments. Under these, market borrowing may be either through direct market access (such as municipal bonds) or from commercial financial intermediaries (Box 11.1).

Most conventional infrastructure investments in other sectors have been developed through a project finance framework, under which new investments generate adequate net returns to ensure a commercial rate of return on investments and it is expected that user fees or charges will be sufficient to generate the necessary revenues.

Box 11.1: Market Access for Financing Water and Sanitation Investments

Developed under the Indo-US Financial Institutions Reform and Expansion (FIRE) Project in 1996, accessing the market for financing urban water and sanitation has caught on in the country. The advantages of market access are ushering in fiscal discipline in operations of the service delivery, additional financing sources, and creation of incentives for better performance. Ahmedabad Municipal Corporation was the first to access the capital market through the issue of municipal bonds in 1998. Since then, 12 more municipal bond issues aggregating to Rs. 12,700 million (US $270 million) have been issued. The GoI provided an impetus to this process through tax exemption for municipal bonds in 1999.

However, direct market access will be applicable only for large cities. Small and medium cities will need to pool their issues to attract capital and reduce the transaction costs. Based on the experience of the US Municipal Bond Market, USAID and the FIRE Project have promoted the concept of Pooled Finance. The first pooled deal concerned 14 small cities in Tamil Nadu, with credit enhancement through a Development Credit Authority (DCA) guarantee from USAID. The second pooled finance deal is expected to take place shortly, providing eight cities in the Bangalore Metropolitan Area in Karnataka with a similar type of credit. Meanwhile, the Indian Government is in the process of establishing a Pooled Finance Development Fund at the national level to provide support to states for credit enhancement and grants for reforms. The case for a pooled finance framework for peri-urban and semi-urban settlements is also strong, as demonstrated in Tamil Nadu and Karnataka.

Currently, the policy at national and state levels for rural water supply included the provision of 90 per cent subsidy for capital investments. It is possible that the remaining portion that is to be contributed by the community will be generated from the pooled finance framework. However, considering the level of subsidy and size of the water and sanitation investments in the rural sector, it may take decades for rural Panchayats to effectively borrow from the market unless the subsidy is reduced substantially and there is ability to pay at the local level.

The first project under the overall FIRE Project, the Tirupur Area Development Project, is developed according to this framework. However, over time, an additional approach has also emerged based on an analysis of finances of several municipal authorities in the country. In cases where a local authority has a relatively strong and stable finance base and performance, even though the net operating revenues from the water/sewerage sector are inadequate to fund the required investments, the projects have been structured within an urban finance framework. Such projects are financed not only on the basis of project revenues, but also on the basis of transfers of net surpluses from other municipal revenues and specific earmarked revenues. Other resources, e.g. from land development, are also used to ensure an adequate rate of return on investments.

This approach is justifiable on the grounds of high economic rates of return generally associated with urban environmental infrastructure projects, although due to the historically low tariff levels the financial rates of return based on sector revenues tend to be low. High economic returns are due to considerable public health and other positive externalities associated with these projects. The urban finance approach needs to be combined with gradual tariff reforms, so that over time it becomes possible to improve the overall financial viability of the sector. Commercial viability within this framework is ensured by an acceptable minimum debt service coverage ratio (>1.33) and security arrangements which may include a trustee-monitored escrow project fund, performance-linked covenants related to total investments by the municipal authorities, debt service reserve funds and market-based financial guarantees. Within this approach, it is essential that overall city-level infrastructure planning and prioritization take place across services to develop a capital investment plan for the overall infrastructure requirements.

PAST AND ON-GOING URBAN SECTOR REFORMS

Following the liberalization by the Government of India and the decentralization ushered in under the 74th Constitutional Amendment Act (CAA) in 1992, the mid-1990s were quite heady days. The enthusiasm for innovation in the urban sector was high and the cities responded wonderfully. Past and on-going reforms in the sector are summarized below.

Management and revenue enhancements at city level: In a number of cases, the revenue base was enhanced through property tax reforms, moderate revision of water charges, improvement of billing and collection, commercial property development, and so on. Attempts have also been undertaken to improve service delivery to the urban poor (Box 11.2). Accounting reforms have taken place in cities in Tamil Nadu, Karnataka (Bangalore) and Maharashtra. In Maharashtra, Environmental Status Reports and Annual Subsidies Reports have been prepared. Community participation has been undertaken through civic services for solid waste management and slum improvement. In Bangalore, the corporate sector participated in the improvement of urban management. In Hyderabad, Chennai and other cities, the amount of unaccounted for water has been reduced.

Box 11.2: Improved Access of Services for the Urban Poor

Models for enhanced services to the urban poor are gradually emerging in the country. They include demand creation and institutionalization of city-wide strategies in Ludhiana and Sangli, slum-networking programme in Ahmedabad, integration of services for the poor within water and sanitation projects such as the Tirupur Area Development Project and subsidized entry fees as practiced in Bangalore. In the case of Ludhiana and Sangli, the FIRE Project in association with Cities Alliance is supporting the city government to create demand for and institutionalize the improvement of service delivery at the city level. In Ludhiana, a three-track approach is planned to network poor settlements to the city within the framework of commercially viable projects (Khosla and Vaidya, 2003) consisting of:

- Improvement of basic service provision through mobilization and organization of communities in underserved settlements including their economic empowerment, awareness building and establishment of linkages with ULBs and other government departments;
- Support to the development of processes and procedures in the ULBs, building of staff capacity and commitment to respond to demands for service provision in presently under-served communities; and
- Encouragement and facilitation of convergence of resources under various relevant state and Central Government programmes and cost contributions from communities to finance the required infrastructure provision in underserved settlements and address critical issues such as land tenure and decentralized management.

In the case of Ahmedabad, the municipal corporation has been implementing a Slum Networking Project in several settlements with the partnership of communities and contributions from industry groups. The corporation has been playing a proactive role in developing these partnerships and streamlining and simplifying procedures for implementation of community-level projects. The corporation is currently in the process of scaling up of this activity to all low-income settlements in the city.

In the case of Tirupur, the New Tirupur Area Development Corporation (NTADCL) is implementing a major water and sewerage project with private sector participation for industrial and domestic users. Within this project, there is a component of subsidized water and sanitation facilities in low-income settlements in municipal areas. The principles of cost recovery are likely to vary for poor households with a subsidy.

In the case of Bangalore, the Bangalore Water Supply and Sewerage Board (BWSSB) completely subsidizes the access charges for the urban poor and is moving towards individual facilities in the case of water supply. The consumption charges remain the same for all users in the city.

Private sector participation: There are as many as 44 initiatives in 25 cities to attract some form of private sector participation in water and sewerage. As many as 55 cities have attempted private sector participation mainly in solid waste disposal through waste-to-compost and waste-to-energy technologies on BOT basis following the Supreme Court of India's intervention. Approximately, 35 such initiatives are operational and the remaining projects are under development. Finally, the introduction of annual service contracts, primarily for labour for water, sewerage and solid waste, followed from the ban on new recruitment by state governments in several cities.

Municipal bonds and credit rating: Initiated under the FIRE Project, 10 large cities have accessed the capital market through municipal bonds. Approximately, 30 cities have undertaken credit rating exercise. In November 2002, Tamil Nadu successfully completed the market borrowing for 14 small and medium towns through pooled finance framework with the support from the USAID DCA Credit Guarantee. Similar initiative for water and sewerage project for eight small and medium cities is proposed in Karnataka.

State-level initiatives: The state of Tamil Nadu has taken the lead in facilitating market-based financing through financial intermediary, municipal bonds and state pooling arrangements. With support from the World Bank, the state is also undertaking substantial capacity building in the sector. It also introduced accounting reforms in all 109 local bodies of the state.

In association with the Department for International Development (DFID) of the UK, the State of Andhra Pradesh is implementing a far-reaching Andhra Pradesh Urban Services for the Poor Project (APUSP). The project aims at a bottom-up approach and municipal reforms, with the objective of achieving sustainable service delivery to all, including the poor, in 32 towns.

The State of Maharashtra has undertaken a very comprehensive review of the urban water sector in consultation with stakeholders. With support from the FIRE project, it has developed recommendations for sector development under its Sukthankar Committee (Government of Maharashtra, 2000). It also restructured the Capital Grants Programme to create incentives for efficiency improvements in the water sector and to introduce private sector participation. Finally, the state prepared a draft note for an independent regulatory framework for water and wastewater and worked on implementing large-scale accounting reforms in its cities.

The Government of Karnataka is currently working on the development of an urban water policy and a pooled finance framework for eight cities in Bangalore's metropolitan area. The Government of Gujarat too has prepared a note on regulatory framework for water (TERI, 2002).

Government of India initiative: The GoI has undertaken the following initiatives:

- Formulation of guidelines for property tax reforms in 1996;
- Introduction of tax-free municipal bonds in 1999;
- Establishment of the City Challenge Fund (CCF) with an initial outlay of Rs. 5,000 million (US $106 million) for the period 2002–7, to create incentives for comprehensive reforms with demand-driven approach in larger cities from 2002 onward. The CCF will pay for transaction and transition costs involved in comprehensive urban sector reforms. The CCF is proposed to be operationsalized in 2003;

- Establishment of the Pooled Finance Development Fund (PFDF) with an initial outlay of Rs. 4,000 million (US $85 million) for the period 2002–7 for facilitating market access for small and medium cities through the establishment of a debt service reserve facility and a grant for reforms. The PFDF will be operationalized in 2003 with support from the FIRE Project;
- Introduction of a model modern municipal legislation to facilitate reforms with support from the FIRE Project;
- Preparation of guidelines for private sector participation with support from the Water and Sanitation Program of the World Bank;
- Establishment of the Urban Reform Initiative Fund (URIF) with an outlay of Rs. 5,000 million (US $106 million) for the Tenth Plan period from 2002 to 2007. URIF is being implemented to create incentives for state governments to make the land and housing markets efficient; and
- Creation of an Urban Sanitation Mission (USM) with an outlay of Rs. 20,000 million (US $425 million). The mission has been proposed for supporting cities to implement the GoI Guidelines for solid waste management which are developed at the direction of the Supreme Court of India.

The on-going initiatives, as outlined above, are initial steps in urban sector reforms and have been 'isolated islands of innovations'. They need to be comprehensive and widespread. Apart from restructuring at the city level (either city-wide comprehensive restructuring or sector-specific systemic reform), there is a substantial reform agenda that needs to be undertaken at the state and city levels to facilitate the enhancement of creditworthiness and sustainable service delivery for contribution to creation of world-class urban systems. These are briefly discussed in the final section, after discussing the experiences with private sector participation.

PRIVATE SECTOR PARTICIPATION IN WATER AND SEWERAGE

The efforts at seeking private sector participation (PSP) in urban water supply and wastewater can be divided into two distinct phases. The first phase corresponds to the period from 1994 to 1999 and the second phase corresponds to 2000 to the present.

Phase I (1994-1999)

Following the liberalization by the GoI and the decentralization ushered in under the 74th CAA, the mid-1990s were heady days with unbridled enthusiasm for innovations in the urban sector. The urban water sector followed in the footsteps of the power sector where the focus was on attracting 'capital from the private sector' since resources were not available within the public sector. As many as 25 cities undertook efforts to attract some form of private sector participation during this period (Table 11.3).

Table 11.3: Nature and Status of Private Sector Participation During 1994–9

City	Nature and status of PSP in water and sewerage
1. Tiruppur Tamil Nadu	Industrial and municipal water and sewerage project with 30-year concession. Initiated in 1994 and the Notice to Proceed to contractor was issued in October 2001. Construction is underway.
2. Hyderabad Andhra Pradesh	BOT for Krishna Bulk Water Supply. Initiated in 1995. Abandoned. BOT for sewerage treatment plant. Initiated in 1996. Abandoned.
3. Cochin Kerala	Industrial water supply project. Pre-feasibility conducted in 1996. Bidding process was not initiated.
4. Bangalore Karnataka	BOT project for Cauvery Bulk Water Supply. Initiated in 1997 and abandoned. ROT (Rehabilitation-Operate-Transfer) of existing system. Initiated in 1997 and abandoned. BOT for two sewage treatment plants (two separate projects). Initiated in 1997 and abandoned.
5. Chennai Tamil Nadu	BOT project for Water treatment plant. Initiated in 1997 and abandoned. A few O&M contracts for pumping stations and treatment plants are operational.
6. Goa	BOT for source development and water treatment plant. Initiated in 1997 and abandoned in 1998.
7. Pune Maharashtra	Build-Finance-Transfer (BFT) for water and sewerage system for construction, finance, operations and billing and collection. Initiated in 1997 and cancelled in 1998.
8. Dewas Madhya Pradesh	Long-term concession for industrial and domestic water and wastewater system. Initiated in 1996 and under development.
9. Vishakapatnam Andhra Pradesh	Long-term concession for industrial and domestic water system. Initiated in 1996 and procurement for construction completed in early 2003. Negotiations for financial closure are underway.
10. Nagpur Maharashtra	BOT for water treatment plant, transmission and distribution system. Initiated in 1998 and abandoned in 1998.

11.	Kolhapur Maharashtra	BOT for water, sewerage and solid waste management. Initiated in 1997 and abandoned in 1997. Solid waste management component is under construction through BOT arrangement.
12.	Surat Gujarat	Initiated as long-term concession for water and wastewater in 1998 and abandonec the same year.
13.	Alandur Tamil Nadu	BOT for sewerage treatment plant of 14 years and construction contract for sewerage system. Initiated in 1997 and the contract was awarded in 1999. Construction completed in 2003.
14.	Haldia West Bengal	BOT for water source development. Initiated in 1998 and abandoned.
15.	Four towns in Karnataka	Mysore, Hubli-Dharwad, Managlore and Belgaon. Initiative by Anglian Water International for operations and maintenance with appropriate investments. Initiated in 1998 and abandoned.
16.	Kakinada Andhra Pradesh	Initiative by Northumbrian Lyonnaise International for operations and maintenance with appropriate investments. Initiated in 1998 and abandoned.
17.	Villapur-Cuddapore and other cities Tamil Nadu	Villapur-Cuddapore and other cities water supply project on BOT basis. Four sewerage projects on BOT basis in cities of Pallavaram, Erode, Karur, Tambaram. Documentation initiated in 1997 and under development.
18.	Delhi	BOT project for water treatment plant. Discussion initiated in 1998 and no action.

Source: Mehta, Meera, 'A Review of Public-Private Partnerships in Water and Sanitation in India: A Study for DFID', and information based on discussions, 1999.

However, only a few projects such as Tirupur Water and Sewerage Project, Alandur Sewerage Project and operation and maintenance contracts in Chennai have been successful. The majority of the remaining projects failed for the following reasons:

- Lack of genuine commitment to reforms, as Indian reforms were initiated out of necessity rather than conviction;
- Lack of clarity in scope and framework for PSP (many of the initiatives in the sector are for Build-Operate-Transfer (BOT)-type projects for source development without adequate concern for management improvements for distribution systems and customer service);
- Lack of rigour in project and contract development, including risk management and lack of adequate concern for financial viability;
- Lack of quality support and funding for project development;

- Lack of policy support and an appropriate regulatory framework at higher levels of government;
- Lack of participation and capacity of a wide variety of stakeholders;
- Lack of continuity of champions for the projects when leaders got transferred or defeated in elections;
- Lack of broad ownership for the project within the city;
- Strong opposition from the existing rent seeking elements who felt threatened.

Innovations during 2000–3: There has been a change of mindset in the sector during the last three years because of lessons learnt during the previous efforts. There is now a widespread consensus on the need to concentrate on the distribution system and service quality of water supplies rather than only on capacity augmentation as attempted during the earlier phase. There is also a gradual emergence of a focus on institutional restructuring to separate the roles of policy, regulations and operations in order to bring in a consumer and commercial orientation. There is an amazing amount of convergence of views on what needs to be done, but with very little urgency on the action front. Table 11.4 presents the on-going efforts, some of which represent the changing focus in the sector.

During this phase, the central government and a few state governments have taken several initiatives to develop an appropriate policy framework and incentive structure for water sector reforms in the country. As discussed above, the GoI has announced setting up of a City Challenge Fund for creating incentives for reforms in the sector and establishing a GoI/state-level pooled finance mechanism for financing urban infrastructure in small and medium towns with support of the FIRE Project, and has taken steps for starting a debate on a regulatory framework for water.

The State of Maharashtra has undertaken a very comprehensive review of the sector in consultation with stakeholders and has developed recommendations for the development of the sector under its Sukthankar Committee. It has also restructured the Capital Grants Programme covering 30 per cent of the state grants, to create incentives for efficiency improvements such as the reduction of unaccounted for water and savings in energy. It has also issued

Table 11.4: Nature and Status of On-going Private Sector Participation Efforts*

	City	Nature and Status of PSP
1.	Bangalore Karnataka	Management contract initiated in early 2001 for two pilot areas of 1 million people each. The contract covers operation and maintenance to improve the service quality and efficiency. Vivendi and Northumbrian Lyonnaise International have jointly submitted a proposal in 2001. Negotiations in 2002. Negotiations collapsed in 2003.
2.	13 towns in Karnataka	Proposal for management contract for O&M in 13 towns. Initiated by the Government of Karnataka in 1999 with support of the World Bank. Under preparation. Down-sized to three cities in 2003. Procurement to begin shortly.
3.	Mumbai Maharashtra	Proposal for management contract for O&M in pilot area with 1 million people. Initiated in early 2000 and under preparation.
4.	Sangli Maharashtra	Proposal for a management contract in Phase I and a concession in Phase II. Initiated during 2000 with support of the Government of Maharashtra, IL&FS and the FIRE Project. Procurement initiated in 2002. Cancelled in January 2003.
5.	Hyderabad Andhra Pradesh	Proposal for either institutional restructuring along the lines of Johannesburg or a concession along the lines of Manila. Initiated in June 2001 with support from the WSP.
6.	Greater Noida Uttar Pradesh	A seven-year O&M contract for water and sewerage with an investment proposal for a sewage treatment plant. Under development since 2002 with support from Feedback Ventures Ltd.
7.	Jamshedpur Jharkhand	Initiative in 2001 by Vivendi for a management contract for the industrial township. Vivendi signed a two-year agreement for the preparatory phase.
8.	Zahirabad Andhra Pradesh	BOT for the entire system. Initiated in 2001 and under development with the support from the HMWSSB.
9.	Delhi Jal Board	Water treatment plant with a 10-year O&M contract awarded in 2001.
10.	Navi-Mumbai Maharashtra	The city had several annual service contracts for water and sewerage, primarily in the form of labour contracts. Moving towards three year consolidated performance contracts. Procurement is underway. Awarding was expected in 2003.
11.	Bangalore Karnataka	Leakage detection and reduction for a pilot area was awarded to Thames Water and L&T in April 2003.

Note: * Other than on-going efforts mentioned in Table 11.3.
Source: Information based on discussions.

guidelines for private sector participation and prepared a draft note on an independent regulatory framework for water and wastewater. The Government of Karnataka is currently working on the development of an urban water policy. The Government of Gujarat has initiated work on a regulatory framework. Even during the current phase, there are not many successful cases for attracting private sector participation at the city level with the possible exception of Navi-Mumbai and Bangalore.

WHAT NEEDS TO BE DONE?

During the next two to three years, it is essential that the focus is on the development of projects to demonstrate commercial market borrowing, institutional restructuring at the local level to create a consumer and commercial orientation, and private sector participation. As far as private sector participation is concerned, it is essential to continue to explore avenues in management with measures to reduce the transaction costs, alternative models consisting of consolidating existing annual service contracts into performance-based annual contracts, promotion of local industry capacity to reduce costs of private sector participation, and utility-to-utility partnerships akin to twinning arrangements in other countries. Only successful demonstration projects will pave the way for major reforms in the country.

In addition, there is a large agenda that remains to be attended to at the state and city levels. The core of the unfinished agenda relates to governance reforms primarily at city and state levels. Unless and until we address the core issue of governance aimed at accountability in public systems, it will not be possible to have comprehensive and widespread reforms in the country. What is necessary is public sector reforms at local and state levels in order to initiate and sustain widespread and sustainable reform processes in the urban sector. The unfinished agenda mainly includes:

- Institutional restructuring to create autonomous and accountable utilities to bring in a consumer and commercial orientation;
- Shifting the focus of urban local bodies from being providers to facilitators and restructuring of state-level water and sewerage boards;
- Enhancement of creditworthiness of cities through innovative resource mobilization, and reducing expenditure responsibilities in favour of private sector involvement and efficiency improvements;

- Restructuring of existing financing arrangements in favour of market-based instruments and incentive and performance-based transfers;
- Establishment of transition management funds by the state and central government to smooth the pain of the reforms;
- Labour reforms including setting of safety nets;
- Development/restructuring of state and national programmes for scaling-up of demand-driven approaches for enhancement of services to the urban poor;
- Setting up of independent regulatory frameworks for water supply and waste water removal, treatment and recycling;
- Simplification or modification of municipal legislations to create downward accountability and facilitate reforms;
- Genuine decentralization ('letting go' of cities) and matching functional responsibility with fiscal autonomy; and
- Development of state or national level support framework for capacity building for reforms at the city level.

One of the key instruments of change relates to the setting up of an independent regulatory framework for water and wastewater at state level to regulate all service providers, including the public sector. The primary objectives will be to improve the service quality, protect the consumers from abuse by the utilities, ensure sustainability of the service and create a conducive environment for investments. Its establishment will serve as a catalyst for reforms by removing the arbitrariness in setting tariffs and service standards and promoting new sector investments. It will also help bring in transparency, accountability and consumer orientation among the sector institutions. The governments of Maharashtra and Gujarat have initiated a dialogue on this framework.

Underpinning this unfinished agenda is the creation of a leadership with courage and conviction to initiate and sustain the reform agenda. In the past, far too many initiatives have failed for lack of good leadership at critical times. It is also essential to create citizen awareness through campaigns, communication and consultation, and foster partnerships with civil society on a large scale.

In conclusion, India and its cities have initiated several positive steps during the last decade. They have provided valuable lessons for furthering sector reforms. Regarding operationalization, the recent initiatives of the national government should create an impetus for the deepening and broadening of reforms in the country. It is essential to consolidate the successes and lessons from failures and foster a greater urgency to act. All of us who are involved in the sector need to make a concerted effort in moving from intended action and debate to action at the earliest. Then and then only will India be able to provide its citizens with sustainable and affordable water and wastewater services in a foreseeable future.

REFERENCES

GoI, *Census of India*, Tables on Houses, Household Amenities and Assets, Series No. 1, New Delhi: Government of India, 2003.

Devi, Kirti and V. Satyanarayana, 'Finances, Resources and Private Sector Participation in Solid Waste Management', paper prepared for Technology Advisory Group (mimeo), New Delhi: Ministry of Urban Development, 2002.

EGCIP, 'The India Infrastructure Report', New Delhi: Expert Group on Commercialization of Infrastructure Projects, Ministry of Finance, Government of India, also Known as Rakesh Mohan Committee Report, 1997.

FIRE Project, 'Various Project Notes', available at www.niua.org.

Government of Maharashtra, 'Sukthankar Committee Report for Water and Sewerage', Mumbai, 2000.

Khosla, Renu and Vaidya Chetan, 'Creating Space for the Poor in Bankable Urban Water Supply and Sewerage Infrastructure Projects', in A. Ghosh (ed.), *Urban Environment Management Local Government and Community Action*, New Delhi: Concept Publishing Co. for Institute of Social Studies and Friedrich Ebert Stiftung, 2003.

Mehta, Meera, 'A Review of Public-Private Partnerships in Water and Sanitation in India', New Delhi: Department for International Development (DFID), 1999.

Mehta, Meera and V. Satyanarayana, 'Commercial Viability in Urban Infrastructure Development in India: From Projects to Institutional Reforms', paper presented at the International Seminar on Financing and Pricing of Urban Infrastructure, New Delhi: Housing and Urban Development Corporation, 8–10 February 1999.

Tata Energy Research Institute, 'Regulatory Framework for Water for Gujarat', New Delhi: TERI, 2002.

CHAPTER 12

Delegating Water Resources Management Issues in Europe: Parallels with India

MEINE PIETER VAN DIJK

INTRODUCTION

This paper gives an impression of water issues in the Netherlands and Germany, based on the impact of the implementation of the European policy in the Drinking Water and Sanitation sector. No original data were collected, but use has been made of publications and review articles in professional journals, listed in the list of references at the end of this paper. The paper describes and analyses developments and notes parallels with water resources management issues in India.

EVALUATION

The water and sanitation sector in the EU member states is most comprehensively covered by European Union directives and the Union's environmental policy. The original series of directives intended to protect the health of the European Union citizens and later efforts were made to harmonize environmental rules in the common market. The assessment of the implications of European Union directives and their implementation at the national level in the case of Germany and the Netherlands is complicated given the piecemeal evolution of legislation over time. Through an intense political process, the directives for water and sanitation have been discussed and accepted in and by the European Institutions, in which issues were dealt with on a problem by problem basis. This process led, according to Kallis and Nijkamp (1999), to a complex picture of water-related directives with differing and often conflicting methodologies, definitions and aims.

In Europe there is also a trend to delegate tasks to a layer of government that is as close as possible to the public at large. In the European context the principle of subsidiarity is used, meaning that activities should be undertaken and decisions be made at the lowest possible level if this is efficient. The idea is that decentralized decision-making institutions can considerably contribute to achieving sustainable water management. Decentralized decision-making institutions require adequate capacity building efforts and the use of integrated water resource management principles in the same management area, such as recovery of cost for water services and the user pays and the polluter pays principles. Users are involved and can participate. Although participation is currently lower than it used to be, the system is still democratic and allows participation.

The European Union directives on drinking water are summarized in Table 12.1. A more detailed description can be found in Annexure 1 of the report of the EU water liberalization study team.

Table 12.1 mainly registers the name of the relevant council directive, gives a short description and the way one commonly refers to these directives.

Table 12.1: Relevant Directives in the Drinking Water Sector

Council directive	Description	Abbreviation
75/440/EEC of 16-6-1975	Quality required of surface water intended for drinking	CD 75/440
76/160/EEC	Quality of bathing water	Bathing water directive
76/464/EEC	Pollution caused by dangerous substances discharged	Dangerous substances
78/659/EEC	Fresh water needing protection for fish life	Fresh water directive
79/923/EEC	Quality required of shellfish waters	Shellfish directive
80/778/EEC of 15-7-1980	Quality of water for human consumption	CD 80/778
91/127/EEC of 1991	Urban wastewater treatment directive	Wastewater treatment
98/83/EC of 3-11-1998	Quality of water intended for human consumption	CD 98/83 or Third Drinking Water Directive
2000/60/EC of 2000	Water framework directive	WFD

The various objectives and topics of European water and sanitation policy have been brought together in the new European Union Water Framework Directive which has been evaluated by Kallis and Nijkamp (1999), Boymans (2002) and Kraemer (2000). The problem is that it is a bit early to assess the impact of the Water Framework Directive in place since 2000 on different European countries. Such an assessment would also require a detailed examination of the complex interplay between issues and actors at the European level and how the results of it are reflected in the chosen regulatory framework (see Box 12.1).

Monitoring and reporting on the implementation of the EU directives has only started after the rules and procedures for it were

Box 12.1: Water Framework Directive

Following the urban wastewater and nitrate directives, new proposals by the European Commission concerned a revision of the standards for bathing and drinking water in 1994, a new directive on the ecological quality of water (1993) and a revision of the process for the deadlocked discharges directive. However, the discussion started whether an integrated approach would not be desired, aiming to integrate all requirements for water management in one single system. This system would be in the river basin and experience was gained through successful programmes in which Germany (and/or the Netherlands) was involved: the management of the Maas, Schelde and Rhine rivers.

The resulting Water Framework Directive has as the guiding goal the achievement of a good status of ground and surface water after about a decade. Good means that water meets the standards established in existing environmental protection directives, in combination with new ecological standards.[1] Important aspects of the WFD are:

- River basin management;
- Cost recovery of water services;
- Participation of all stakeholders in relevant decisions;
- Reporting (i.e. the implementation process and effects); and
- Protection of groundwater and wetlands.

For countries receiving water from upstream neighbours, such as Germany and the Netherlands, potential gains of the Water Framework Directive are expected from a better water quality policy upstream.

subsequently laid down in a number of separate directives. The evidence concerning the shortcomings in the implementation of the first directives has mounted the calls for a reconsideration of approaches:

> The need to take integrated action for protecting the Union's waters, both for human and environmental purposes, was raised at various European fora. At the same time, Member States, realising the costs involved in achieving the environmental and public health objectives of the directives and meeting local difficulties in applying European Union wide regulations, have stressed the need for a decentralised, simplified and economically viable approach. (Kallis and Nijkamp, 1999)

IMPACT OF EUROPEAN LEGISLATION ON THE GERMAN WATER AND SANITATION SECTOR

The future poses significant challenges for the German water and sanitation sector: (i) rising sea levels, (ii) an expected subsidence of the surface, (iii) climatological changes, (iv) increasing urbanization, and (v) the requirement to comply with stringent European legislation standards for wastewater treatment, laid down in the Urban Waste-water Treatment Directive. Especially the removal of nitrogen will necessitate Germany to make big investments in the coming years. Financing these additional investments is likely to follow the same 'rules' as have been implemented for many decades in the water sector in Germany. If this is not sufficient, additional funds will have to be made available to live up to the Wastewater Treatment Directive.

The German model is a decentralized system often initiated by private initiative of the stakeholders. It is characterized by Kraemer (2002: 329) as the model maintaining competition in the water industry and democratic control through municipalities. He considers the model similar to the one used in the Netherlands. The main characteristics are summarized in Box 12.2.

The current German debate concerns the conditions under which the private sector can participate in the water and sanitation sector (Hansen et al., 2001). The debate focusses on the consequences that a different structure in the water sector could have on the environment and water management. More regulation is seen as the natural counterpart of privatization and would concern more transparency

Box 12.2: The German Model in the Water Sector

- It is not regulatory in the usual sense of the word of an external regulatory authority and the private operator of the utility. Influence is exercised through ownership rights and municipal authorities involved in the operation of urban water services.
- The operation of water systems is strictly separated from the production and provision of most water-related goods and services to limit the risk of inefficiencies.
- Competition exists in all segments of the water industry, except for the municipal agency or enterprise established to operate natural monopolies.
- Inter-municipal associations have been established for the purpose of supplying water.
- The model builds on a tradition of municipal autonomy and efficient provision of public services.

Source: Kraemer (2000).

and control, benchmarking, liability, price regulation, health and environmental considerations.

For the first key directive of 1975 (COM 75 440), Germany had extensive legislation for the functioning of the municipalities and the municipal enterprises as joint stock companies (AG) or partnerships with limited liability (GmbH), and, therefore, the directive did not change the practice of supplying water very much. It mainly contributed to the notion that such matters are no longer national or (Bundes) State issues but have become European Union responsibilities.

In 1976, the European Union dealt with the quality of water and regulated in particular the discharge of dangerous substances into the aquatic environment (COM 76 464). The underlying principles were that water use directives concerned with the quality of water are standards for the all of Europe and are to be complied with by all member states, while water pollutant directives, concerned with the control of emissions of particular pollutants to water, are setting emission standards to be respected in all member states (Somsen, 1990). This directive is not a great problem for Germany, since the country, contrary to some other European countries, has followed an emission control approach for a long time under the Regulation of

Matters Relating to Water of 1957 (Federal Water Act WHG), last amended in 2001, as a framework law of the Federal Government that lays down basic provisions relating to the management of water quality and quantity.

The directive relating to the quality of water intended for human consumption and the water in the distribution system is considered the second drinking water directive (CD 80/778), which has been revised by COM 98 83, which we call the third drinking water directive (CD 98/83). This can be called for short the water standards to be respected 'at the tap'. Subsequently Germany established parameters for the waters concerned, which were no less stringent than the mandatory values and try to respect the stricter values (Howarth, 1992). Germany had to prepare an integrated programme for the reduction of their emissions of List II substances in COM 80 68.

The Urban Wastewater Treatment Directive of 1991 aimed at the collection, treatment and discharge of sewage from urban centres and specified industrial sectors (COM 91 271). Implementation of this directive required heavy investments in most countries and some cities (in particular Brussels and Milan) announced they would not be able to meet the official deadline. Kallis and Nijkamp (1999) consider the huge financing of construction works necessary to comply with the directive to provide a further push for organizational restructuring of water management and the full or partial privatization of the water industry. This is certainly the case in Germany as well as the Netherlands, although water companies that had developed sufficient sewage control systems were found to be in a comparatively better position than those with no developed structures.

Germany tends to be ahead of other European Union countries as can be seen in the case of the nitrate directive, where it was one of the only five countries which had established a genuine action programme (CEC, 1997).

CONCLUSIONS FROM THE GERMAN CASE STUDY

Germany is a typical example of a state with a well-developed environmental legislation. This means the country can afford to push for stricter environmental rules, on the one hand because of domestic pressure, and on the other hand to create a level playing field.

Secondly, Germany, with countries like Spain would want less power at the European Union to regain control over various policies. Subsidiarity is considered important in order to maintain the autonomous character of their regions (Kallis and Nijkamp, 1999). The Netherlands welcomes it for the reason that it allows the country to continue with respect to the distinctive system that it has put in place in the course of at least ten centuries.

However, it is also noted that Germany, in the past a fast mover in the field of environmental policy, after the unification of East and West Germany and the emerging problems with its economy has become more inward looking.

The improvements in the German water and sanitation sector could be attributed to increasingly stringent controls of water quality between 1986 and 1993 initiated by European legislation but also by additional measures taken by the competent authorities in the member states. It certainly helped that Germany now had to report its activities in this field to a higher European arbiter. As Kallis and Nijkamp (1999) phrase it: 'The setting of legally-enforceable water quality standards and the public availability of information on the compliance with such standards have opened the administrative structures, leading to a greater flow of information regarding pollution and quality of the aquatic environment.'

Contrary to countries like the UK and Italy, Germany did not have to do huge investments to comply with these directives. In the UK it added to the drive for private sector involvement in the water sector, which was not the case in Germany in the 1980s.[2] Germany, like the Netherlands, also had the administrative and monitoring structures in place for water management and hence found it relatively easy to comply with the European Union directives.

IMPACT OF EUROPEAN LEGISLATION ON THE DUTCH SECTOR

Since the beginning of water supply provision in the Netherlands in the 1850s, the sector has evolved continuously. This evolution is illustrated by the various modes of organization that have been dominant since the first water supply company started operating in 1853. From 1853–1920, water supply provision was largely a private enterprise in which privately owned companies provided potable water to customers. Partly because of these early 'private' beginnings, the water supply sector has always had a history of full-cost recovery. In the period between 1921–74, in which the importance of safe water supply was fully realized, the municipal public utilities became the predominant mode of water services delivery. From 1975 onwards, the government-owned public limited company became the most prominent mode of organization for supplying potable water. The prominence of the public water PLC resulted largely from government regulation, most notably the Drinking Water Supply Act and amendments to this Act in 1975, which promoted the '[a]malgamation of water utilities into larger vertically integrated units under the public water PLC format', whilst 'horizontal integration with other utilities and other institutional forms were discouraged' (Blokland et al., 2000). The number of water supply companies, which are only responsible for production and/or distribution of potable water, dropped from 210 in 1950 to 15 at present (VEWIN, 2002).

The essence of the government-owned PLC is that the company is established and operates under Company Law whilst the shares of the company are in hands of national, regional or local government authorities. Generally, there is no legal or organizational difference between a publicly-owned and a privately-owned PLC apart from the government ownership of shares (Schwartz and Blokland, 2002). The implication is financial transparency. This may not be enough, however, to guarantee economic efficiency. For that reasons, the sector implemented self-regulation in 1989 through annual performance comparison. The idea is to develop it into a full-fledged benchmarking system, creating a surrogate market in the otherwise monopolistic business of piped water supply. The annual reports that they have to publish serve as the basis for the banks to assess the creditworthiness of individual utilities and to determine their credit ceilings. In fact, the banking sector, together with central government pushes the utilities towards performance comparison, rather than compliance with any EU directive.

The distribution of tasks and responsibilities in the water sector in the Netherlands is largely historically defined. History has resulted in a fragmentation of responsibilities over a multitude of actors as shown in Table 12.2. Strategic and operational policy is formulated at four

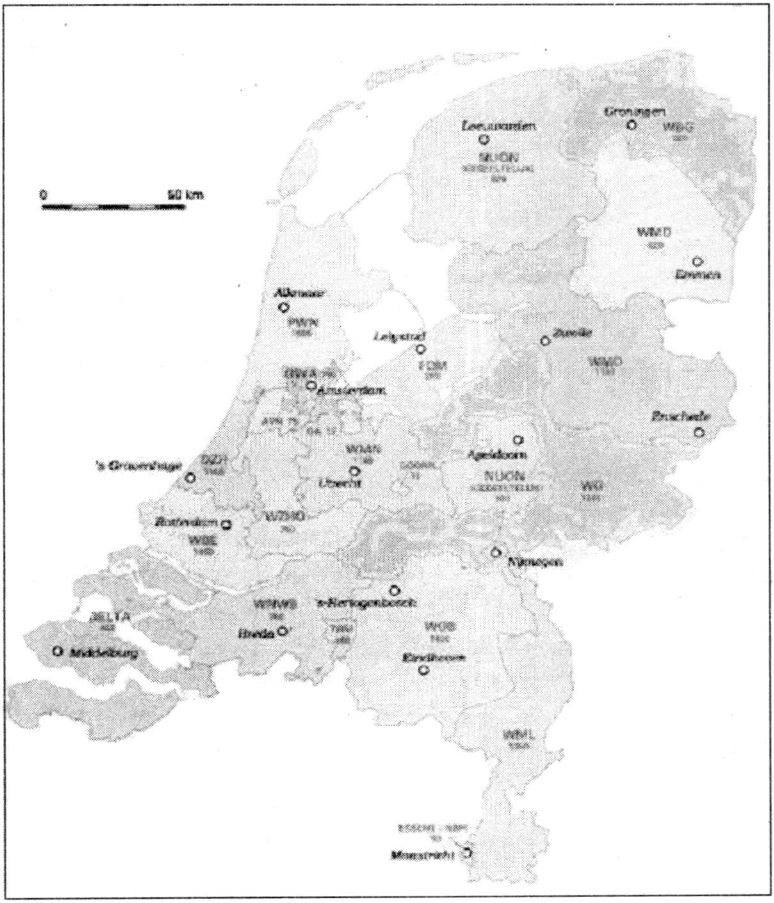

Source: H2O.

Figure 12.1: The Dutch Water Supply Companies

different levels of government involving no less than seven different institutions. Responsibilities concerning water policy formulation are attributed to the European Union, the central government, the provincial government, the municipal government, the water boards, the Netherlands Waterworks Association (VEWIN), and the individual drinking water companies.[3] Table 12.2 summarizes the current distribution of responsibilities in the water sector in the Netherlands over the major actors.

Table 12.2: Water Activities in the Public Sector in the Netherlands

Activity	Responsible organization	Major source of finance
Flood control	National government/Water boards	Govt. budget/taxation
Water quality management	Water boards	WB charge/pollution levy
Water supply management	Water companies	Tariffs/capital market
Wastewater collection	Municipalities and Water boards	Municipal taxes/WB charges
Water treatment	Water boards financing	Capital market/project

The increasing number of directives and their implications has led water boards and water companies in the Netherlands to increasingly use consultants to help them apply these regulations. This trend is reinforced by the drive for more efficiency in the nineties, which led many water companies to doing away with staff departments and hire consultants instead.

Besides the European Union directives, different levels of government in the Netherlands also influence the water sector (Table 12.3). It is important to analyse the role of different stakeholders, in particular if they have different interests. In the Netherlands local governments do not allow individual farmers or companies to treat their wastewater if there are collective systems nearby, because the individual action could go at the expense of the collective efforts.

The Dutch have a long tradition of managing water. The fact that water management is an expensive business can be illustrated by pointing to the experience in the Netherlands. Water control activities alone in this country cost US $386 per inhabitant in 1994. These total cost are made up of flood protection cost (16 per cent), cost for water quantity control (19 per cent) and for water quality control (65 per cent).

According to the Surface Water Pollution Act, charges are being levied in order to finance water quality management, including wastewater treatment. As such, the expenditure on water quality is covered completely through the pollution levy. The pollution levy is based on a 'pollution unit', which is equivalent to the amount of wastewater one person produces per year. In 1999, the average

Table 12.3: Overview of Responsibilities in the Dutch Water Sector

Organization	Responsibility
Central Government	Framework acts and general administrative measures Strategic national policy Operational policy and management for the North Sea and national water systems General supervision over provinces, water boards and municipalities
Provinces	Strategic groundwater and surface water policy Operational groundwater policy and management General supervision over water boards and municipalities.
VEWIN	Draft 10-year plans every 5 years
Water boards	Surface water management (quantity and quality), water control, management of inland waterways and some small inland roads
Municipalities	Sewerage collection
Drinking water companies	Production and distribution of drinking water Draft one-year plans

Source: Based on Mostert, 1997.

pollution levy was € 41.7 per 'pollution unit'. A family on average pays for three pollution loads or € 125.2 per year (Union of Water Boards, 2002). The amount levied per pollution load ranges between different water boards from almost € 50 to € 32. The difference in levy is closely linked to the costs for treating wastewater.

For industries tailormade approaches are in operation. Industrial levies are based on the quantity and substance of their wastewater. Eighty per cent of the income generated by the pollution levy is spent on wastewater treatment. The remaining 20 per cent is spent on other activities aimed at improving the quality of surface waters (Union of Water Boards, 2001). The total costs for water management in the Netherlands amount to € 5.67 billion per year (Ministry of Transport and Public Works, 2000). More than half of this amount goes to water supply provision and water quality management. The water boards collect the water board charges and pollution levy. The water supply companies collect the drinking water charges. Financing of water management activities derives from six sources:

- Central Government budget
- Water board charge
- Pollution levy
- Groundwater taxes

- Drinking water charges
- Private project financing

In the year 2000, the average total cost per water connection in the Netherlands was € 205 per connection (VEWIN, 2001). These are the average cost per connection. Between water supply companies the costs per connection fluctuates strongly from € 241 per connection for one of the companies using surface water to € 147 for one of the companies using groundwater as a main water source (VEWIN, 2001). With over 7 million connections in 2000 (VEWIN, 2002), the total costs in the water sector approximate € 1.4 billion. Of the total expenditure in the water supply sector, approximately half is operational cost (47 per cent), 10 per cent is taxes, 22 per cent is capital costs and a further 21 per cent is depreciation (VEWIN, 2001). Over the past decade the total investments in the Dutch water supply sector have averaged around € 500 million per year. In 2000 investments reached € 419 million, which represents € 28 per inhabitant. Most of the investments went into distribution (50 per cent), 39 per cent in production processes and about 4 per cent in information and communication technology (VEWIN, 2002).

The water supply sector finds itself in an era in which investments are likely to increase substantially over the coming decades. The expected increase in required investments is due to a number of factors (Braadbaart and Hoogwout, 1999):

- *Continuing aggregation of companies*: It is expected that the current 15 companies will be subject to future mergers, reducing the total to between 3 and 6. These mergers are likely to involve considerable additional investments.
- *Increasing cost of raw water*: The deteriorating quality and availability of groundwater is likely to drive up treatment costs. On the one hand, groundwater regulation will likely force companies to shift from groundwater to surface water (which requires more extensive treatment), on the other hand, intensive agriculture has polluted groundwater sources and complicated water treatment.
- *Increase in cost of new treatment plants*: New plants tend to be outfitted with costly advanced treatment technologies. This is partly explained by the pollution problems mentioned above

as well as the need to adhere to increasingly stringent environmental procedures.

Finally, a problem that the companies are confronted is with the need to make additional investments to meet increasing stringent water quality and to satisfy environmental management requirements imposed partially by the European Union and partially by the climate and other environmental considerations.

Wastewater treatment is a joint responsibility of the municipalities, which transport it and the water boards that clean it. In 2002, the Water Board Delfland awarded a Design-Build-Finance-Operate (DBFO) contract to the Delfluent Consortium for the construction and operation of one of Europe's largest wastewater treatment plants, which should be operational in 2008 (as well as upgrading an older treatment plant).[4] The concession has a duration of 30 years. The decision to involve the private sector rested on the need to build a new treatment plant (in light of the need to meet EU guidelines on urban wastewater discharge).[5] The Water Board Delfland believes the DBFO scheme will at least provide efficiency gains of 10 per cent.

With the awarding of the first DBFO contract, private sector financing has made its entry into the Dutch water sector. At present, this is the first and only project of its kind. It remains to be seen to what extent private sector financing will grow over the coming decades. In light of the challenges facing the Dutch water sector, however, it is clear that it will definitely be seen as a viable option by many decision makers. The lessons so far are that the process takes more time than expected and that there will be a need to monitor the project to find out whether it achieves its goals.

IMPACT OF EUROPEAN LEGISLATION ON DUTCH LEGISLATION

The first drinking water directives (CD 75/440) are incorporated in the waterworks decision and the decision quality objectives and measurement of surface waters. These laws focus on water use by water companies. The law was changed in 1984 to implement the European Union directives, (including the second drinking water directives: CD 80/778). Boymanns (2002) mentions as the most important effect of this EU directive the replacement of lead tubes. Although replacement started earlier, the EU directive was an extra impulse to finish in time.

The Urban Wastewater Treatment Directive of 1991 is incorporated in the Environmental Management Act ('Wet Milieubeheer') and the act concerning pollution of surface waters ('Wet Verontreiniging van Oppervlaktewater'). Directive 91/676 is incorporated in the Soil Protection Act ('Wet Bodembescherming') and the Nitrate Directive ('Nitraatrichtlijn'). Entire Netherlands was designated as vulnerable zone in 1994. In 1995 an action programme was launched to fulfil the requirements of the directive.

The third drinking water directives (CD 98/83) came at a time when water companies in the Netherlands started experimenting with private sector involvement. However, the government introduced in 2002 a law that will reserve the water sector exclusively for public ownership. The emphasis is on the public water PLC, which is usually government owned, but under private law (Blokland et al., 2000). Instead of real competition, a system of benchmarking was introduced to allow the water companies to compare their performance (VEWIN, 2000, 2001 and 2002).

CONCLUSIONS FROM THE DUTCH CASE STUDY

The Dutch water sector is unique in many ways, as the same sector in any other country is also likely to be unique. The water sector in the Netherlands has largely been defined by cultural and historical traditions, some of which date back to the Middle Ages. Despite this observation some general conclusions can be drawn which may provide valuable lessons for the water sector in other parts of the world. We like to point to the factors that play an important role in the decision-making process about financing water management in the Netherlands.

One of the principles of efficient and sustainable water management in the Netherlands is that stakeholders participate directly or through representation to make good management possible. The functioning of the water boards is based on people's participation and on the 'profit principle' (Huisman, 1997). Who benefits will pay, but also gets a say, or in plain Dutch: 'Wie profiteert betaalt mee, maar betaling geeft zeggenschap.' The Dutch government has made the choice to consider water management a public responsibility, but stimulates water organizations to go for private finance of certain water-related activities (there is, for example, a centre for PPP in the Ministry of Finance). The government is trying to increase the efficiency of the water sector by promoting benchmarking, the achievement of economies of scale and the outsourcing of certain tasks. The supervisory tasks are financed from the general budget. The 'Dutch Model' is characterized by a landscape of financing options. It is left to the managers of the water boards and water supply companies to select the option of financing that best suits their need. Often one company will combine different financing options, depending on what is most suitable for them at a specific moment.

Because of the investments required as mentioned above, water utilities and water boards are more and more dependent on external financiers. However, water supply companies offer attractive prospects for capital investment and this has contributed to the development of a close relationship between Dutch water utilities and financial institutions. Braadbaart and Hoogwout (1999) conclude that because of this water utilities are slowly bringing their financial recording and reporting procedures in line with private sector standards to meet the demands of external financiers. Investors demand transparency in financial matters. For that reason, the Dutch habit of cross-utility performance comparison based on a consistent accounting methodology justifies the considerable effort made to put it in place. Indicators are solvency rates, but performance indicators also play an increasingly important role. Typically most water companies are trying to improve these indicators.

The conclusion concerning the Netherlands case study is summarized in Box 12.4. Given the financial implications of the European directives, private sector participation (PSP) in the water sector is more likely in the future and hence requires more attention. Attracting private capital requires a different approach to water projects. These projects now have to convince financial people that they are worth putting their money into it. This requires an identification of the possible risks (Lindfield, 1998). The increasing role for the private sector institutions and the importance of public

Box 12.4: Factors Explaining the Relative Success of the Dutch Model

The importance of strong financial institutions being present cannot be overstated:

- The authorities have made a conscious choice to go for those organizations falling under public law for the water boards and public ownership for the water companies;
- The role of the bank for the water boards is a prime example of a strong financial institution, which has played a crucial role in the financing of the water sector;
- There is a sense of urgency concerning water management, reinforced by the 1953 floods. It has led to broad support for the activities of water boards and water companies;
- The positive interaction between demand (the water boards and water supply companies) and supply (the financial institutions) on the other hand is very important;
- The water boards and water companies have developed a solid reputation in terms of financial reliability and have built up trust;
- It is a decentralized system often initiated by private initiative and stakeholders;
- The use of integrated water resources management principles such as recovery of cost and the water user pays and the polluter pays' principles;
- Users are involved and can participate;
- The importance of financial reputation–lower levels of government to have a good financial reputation in the Netherlands;
- Creating a special intermediary financial institution like the NWB;
- The current legal framework, for example, does not allow water companies to run deficits; and
- The system of self-regulation of water boards and water companies–benchmarking is undertaken by the sector itself, which makes it possible to detect sources of inefficiency.

private partnerships (PPP) does not mean that the ownership of the water boards or companies has to be private.

GENERAL CONCLUSIONS

From these country experiences it can be concluded that the issues at stake are three fold. One, at what level do we want to regulate the water and sanitation sector. If we follow the subsidiarity principle in this sector, would not a lot more be left to the national, regional and local level? Kallis and Nijkamp (1999: 9–10) review a number of arguments against centralized European approaches to environmental protection and water. They consider the directives have evolved with reference to well-developed administrative and monitoring structures of the more progressive environmental protection states. Development of such structures in the less advanced member countries is slow and often a long-term process.

Secondly, different stakeholders have different interests. In the Netherlands, local government does not allow individual companies to treat their wastewater if there are collective systems, because the individual action could go at the expense of the collective efforts. Also in this sector there is a complex interaction of institutional actors and organizations of concerned individuals. This complicates the formulation of European water policies and makes their implementation even more difficult.

Finally, there may be a conflict between different objectives of the EU, such as the desire to deregulate, the wish to protect the environment and the principle of subsidiarity. The problems in applying these objectives in a coherent way become clear if applied to the major issues in the water and sanitation sector, such as private or public supply, large-scale or small-scale treatment, individual or collective solutions.

Kallis and Nijkamp (1999: 6) draw another important conclusion namely that there is a relation between the nature and the success of a water directive. Directives that tackle sensitive and easily understandable public use of water, such as bathing and drinking water, had a more important impact because of the public attention they generated. Directives with less clear objectives (they give the example of the fish and shellfish directives), which are not as clear whether they serve a public health purpose (or seem to be controlled more easily in a different way, for example, by controlling the quality of the final product in the fish market) do not have the same impact.

Kallis and Nijkamp (1999) also conclude that it is very difficult to draw a conclusion on the effects of the first water directive, which at least triggered off intensive activities in most of the member states, including Germany. However, whether the directives also generated a direct change in the quality of the Union's surface and bathing waters they consider more difficult to assess. Although reduction of concentrations of regulated point source pollutants have been observed in European lakes, rivers and coastal waters, an increase has been observed from unregulated sources according to the European Environmental Agency (EEA, 1995).

The Water Framework Directive is a new stage and is considered a piece of legislation that tries to amend European Union water legislation in the light of the problems that appeared during the application of the previous water legislation (Boymans, 2002: 22). However, he also notes that it leaves more possibilities to the member states concerning the interpretation of the provisions. Member states like the Netherlands and Germany tend to go beyond the minimal requirements set by the water framework directives, while others may take a minimalist approach. In the Netherlands this is certainly not the case.

NOTES

1. A water is defined as of good ecological quality if there is only slight departure from the biological community that would be expected in conditions of minimal anthropogenic impact.
2. An interesting analysis of the process of private sector involvement in the water sector in the UK can be found in the article of Bakker (2003).
3. For the rich history of the water boards we refer to Union of Water Boards (1997), or a CD rom 'Water Boards in the Netherlands', made available by the Union of the Water Boards.
4. The Delfluent Consortium incorporates Vivendi Water, DELTA Water, Water Company Europoort, Rabobank, Heijmans Groundworks and Civil Engineering and Strukton.
5. Different forms of privatization can be distinguished, ranging from complete divestiture to privatizing only certain stages of the production process (van Dijk and Schulte Nordholt, eds., 1994). Only certain functions, such as the management, may be privatized, or certain tasks could be contracted out to private partners. Finally, involvement of the private sector is also possible by using management or service contracts or through concessions. In this case the property is not transferred, but only the management. An early summary of experiences of involving the private sector in the supply of urban services, such as water supply and sewerage can be found in Roth (1989). An example of the latter is the public–private partnership for the water purification plant for the region The Hague.

REFERENCES

ABN-AMRO (1996), De Watersector. Amsterdam: ABN-AMRO Bank.

Bakker, K.J., 'Paying for Water, Water Pricing and Equity in England and Wales', in: Royal Geographical Society, 2001, pp. 134–66.

———, 'From Public to Private to Mutual? Restructuring Water Supply Governance in England and Wales', in *Geoforum*, 2003.

Blokland, M., O. Braadbaart and K. Schwartz. 'The Public Water PLC'. Delft: IHE, 2000.

BNG, Review of Operations, The Hague: Bank of the Dutch Municipalities, 1997.

Boymans, D., European Policies and Sustainable Use of Water in Metropolitan Areas', Seville: IPTS, 2002.

Braadbaart, O. and B.J. Hoogwout, Investment Financing and Cost Recovery: How Water Dompany Oost-Brabant Does it', working paper, Delft: IHE, 1999.

CEC, Fourteenth Annual Report on Monitoring the Application of Community Law (97/C332/01), 1997.

Dijk, M.P. and N.G. Schulte Nordholt, 'Privatisation Experiences in Africa and Asia', Amsterdam: SISWO, 1994.

EEA, 'Europe's Environment, The Dobris Assessment, European Environmental Agency', in D. Stanners and P. Burdeau (eds.), 1995.

Hansen, W., E. Interwies and R.A. Kraemer, 'Privatisierungen der Wasserwirtschaft in Europa', in *GWF Wasser-Abwasser*, vol. 143, no. 8, 2001.

Huisman, P., 'Financing Water Management Cost in the Netherlands', in Van Hofwegen and Schultz (eds.), 1997.

Howarth, W., 'New Strategies for Water Directives', in *European Environmental Law Review*, vol. 1, no. 4, 1992, pp. 117–22.

Kallis, G. and P. Nijkamp, 'Evolution of European Union Water Policy: A Critical Assessment and a Hopeful Perspective', Amsterdam: Free University Research Memorandum 27, 1999.

Kraemer, R.A., 'Public and Private Water Management in Europe', in *Selected Issues in Water Resources Management in Europe*, 2000, pp. 319–52.

Lindfield, M., 'Preparing Markets for Private Financing of Urban Infrastructure', Rotterdam: Erasmus University, Ph.D. thesis, 1998.

Ministry of Transport and Public Works, 'New Deal with an Old Enemy, Water Management in the Netherlands', The Hague: Ministry of Verkeer and Waterstaat, 2000.

Mostert, E., 'Water Policy Formulation in The Netherlands', *Water 21*, Phase 1 report, Research Report nr.6, Delft: RBA, 1997.

Schwartz, K. and M. Blokland, 'Government-owned Public Limited Companies in the Dutch Water Sector: The Case of the Water supply Company Limburg and Water company Europoort', in Seidenstat, P., Haarmeyer, D. and S. Hakim, *Reinventing Water and Wastewater Systems: Global Lessons on Improving Water Management*, New York: John Wiley & Sons, 2002.

Somsen, 'EC Water Directives', in *Water Law*, November 1990.

Union of Water Boards, *Water Boards*, The Hague: Union Waterschappen, 1997.

———, Water Boards in the Netherlands, CD-ROM, The Hague: Union Waterschappen, 2002.

VEWIN, Waterleidingstatistiek 2000, Rijswijk: VEWIN, 2000.

———, Reflections on Performance 2000: Benchmarking in the Dutch Drinking Water Industry, Rijswijk: VEWIN, 20001.

———, http://www.vewin.nl, 2002.

CHAPTER 13

The Water Sector Reform and the Roles for Research

CHRISTINE SIJBESMA AND MEINE PIETER VAN DIJK

WATER AND SANITATION IN A CHANGING ENVIRONMENT

In the past 25 years, India has done very well in improving the access of its population to better drinking water. Coverage went up from 31 per cent in rural areas and 77 per cent in urban areas in 1980 to 80 per cent and 94 per cent in 2000 (Reddy, Ch. 6). Nearly 95 per cent of the rural population has at least one improved source of drinking water. Expansion has been particularly rapid during the water decade when coverage went up from 31 per cent in 1980 to 78 per cent in 1991. India's achievements are also impressive in the global context. In *The Human Development Report* of 1998, the percentage of people without access to an improved drinking water supply was 19 per cent in India as compared to 23 per cent in Latin America, 32 per cent in East Asia, 35 per cent in South-East Asia and the Pacific, and 48 per cent in Sub-Saharan Africa. Factors contributing to this success were the priority to drinking water supply in the national policy, with substantial allocations under consecutive Five Year Plans, and a combination of national and state programmes. Bilateral and international cooperation also played a role (van Dijk and Sijbesma, Ch. 1; Reddy, Ch. 5).

These achievements are under threat. In the first chapter, Nijkamp pointed out that water is an economic good and people need to get used to considering good water supply as something requiring investments that needs to be earned back. Growing competition for, and deteriorating quality of freshwater constitute serious problems for the supply and management of drinking water in many countries. To be delivered in sufficient quantity and with safe quality, this water has to be pumped up from ever increasing depths, transported over ever increasing distances and be treated more thoroughly, which greatly increases its costs. The poor management of water as a basic human resource also affects India the second most populous country in the world.

While increased irrigation coverage has made India self-sufficient in food production, it has also brought new problems: water shortages, lower groundwater levels, soil salination, inequitable water distribution between users, loss of livelihood for displaced people, non-adjustment of irrigation systems to other water uses, and conflicts between Indian states and between India and its neighbours (van Dijk and Sijbesma, Ch. 1). The quality of drinking water is affected negatively by high levels of fluoride and arsenic in groundwater in parts of the country and by the lack of good sanitation for over 80 per cent of the rural and about 25 per cent of the urban population (Reddy and Dev, Ch. 4; Reddy, Ch. 5). This, and the lack of treatment of wastewater and the installation of soak pit latrines in high water table areas cause bacteriological contamination of surface water and shallow groundwater. The contamination and over-extraction of groundwater are of particular concern as groundwater meets 85 per cent of the rural drinking water needs and sustains 60 per cent of the irrigated agriculture (Burjia, Ch. 2).

A further problem is the poor reliability and sufficiency of water deliveries. Under a supply-driven approach, supply suffers from a vicious circle of low tariffs and poor user payments, leading to a lack of resources for adequate maintenance and repairs, a continuing poor service delivery and perennial poor user payments (Sankar, Ch. 3; James and Moriarty, Ch. 10). Water shortages in rural areas range from 4 to 30 per cent and in urban areas from 2 to 30 per cent (Reddy and Dev, Ch. 4).

Achieving coverage for the last 15 per cent in the rural areas and maintaining universal access has proven unexpectedly difficult. In some states, access to improved water supply is less than 50 per cent. Nationwide, 26 per cent of the rural population still relies on open wells (Sankar, Ch. 3) whose hygienical use is unlikely. The figures also leave unaddressed that access refers only to the equation of minimally one improved water point supplying 40 lpcd within a defined reasonable distance (James and Moriarty, Ch. 10) and not to access and use on the ground (Kumar, Ch. 7).

Financially, budget allocations of Rs. 2.5 billion/year for operation and maintenance of the existing water supplies form less than 10 per cent of the estimated actual requirements of Rs. 29 billion. For rehabilitation, repairs and extension to the still unserved areas, the investment requirements is some Rs. 200 billion, of which Rs. 110 billion would be for new construction (Sankar, Ch. 3; Reddy and Dev, Ch. 4). Overall, expenditures of the centre and states have averaged almost Rs. 38 billion per year, which is vastly inadequate to meet the requirements for sustaining existing water supplies and filling gaps. Moreover, the ongoing financing of the water and sanitation sector through plan allocations by the central and state governments has led to a situation of inappropriate incentives, inefficient utilization of funds and widespread service inefficiencies (Satyanarayana, Ch. 11). Allocations to water supply and sanitation in state budgets have more or less stagnated at 7 per cent (Reddy and Dev, Ch. 4).

POWER TO THE PEOPLE AND THEIR ELECTED BODIES

The response of the central government has been to introduce new water policies and programmes. In 2002, the country adopted a revised National Water Policy. It emphasizes the integrated management of all water resources at the basin and sub-basin levels and gives drinking water supply the highest priority for allocation (Burjia, Ch. 2). The policy stresses the involvement of people in project planning and the management of water resources. However, the national law can only give general guidance. Surface water falls under the jurisdiction of the state governments, while groundwater belongs de facto to the owners of the land, which has led to serious depletion and negative impacts for poor people and women relying on public sources. Fragmentation is common and a holistic community approach to water development, use and management within households, communities and watersheds is missing.

The law, for example, advocates including provisions for domestic water use in irrigation schemes only when the communities concerned do not have other sources for drinking water. Nor have drinking water supply activities integrated with water conservation and watershed programmes (Reddy, Ch. 5) been made to involve the private sector in water and sanitation projects. This new approach of increasing private sector participation is suggested in Chapter 1 by van Dijk and Sijbesma, and documented in Chapter 11 by Satyanarayana.

The Panchayat Act of 1992, laid down in the 73rd and 74th Amendments to the Constitution, shifted the responsibilities for water supply and sanitation, along with 27 other responsibilities, from state agencies to local governments. The Acts created the legal opportunity for community-managed water supply and sanitation and public-private partnerships (van Dijk and Sijbesma, Ch. 1; Kumar, Ch. 7; Satyanarayana, Ch. 11).

Government water supply agencies undertook the first pilot projects for community-managed water supply and sanitation with bilateral funding. This was followed by a pilot project in the State of Uttar Pradesh which was executed by a separate project organization and financed by a state loan from the World Bank (Sijbesma, Ch. 8). These initial pilots were followed by a country-wide pilot project planned and financed by the central government and implemented nationwide in 63 districts. In these districts, individual Panchayats could plan, implement and run their own improved community water supplies with 90 per cent direct funding from central government if they contributed 10 per cent of the investment costs and thereafter operated and managed the systems themselves (Kumar, Ch. 7; Shordt, Ch. 9). Before the national pilot project was completed and evaluated, the Indian government upgraded it to a national programme called Swajaldhara (Ministry of Rural Development, 2002).

A companion programme, the Total Sanitation Campaign, is to raise rural latrine coverage to 50 per cent. The programme provides funds for campaigns to raise demand for latrines in rural areas. The demand is met by encouraging the local private sector, NGOs and individual householders to open production centres and shops, and by training local masons on low-cost latrines (Shordt, Ch. 9). Alternatively, Panchayats and water and sanitation committees can plan and implement local programmes for improved sanitation and give subsidies from their own resources to households unable to pay (Sijbesma, Ch. 8; Kumar, Ch. 7).

In urban areas, more efforts have been made to promote private sector participation. India is not the only country that has adopted a strategy of decentralization and devolution for water supply and sanitation and translated it into national programmes. The experiences from these programmes are also relevant for many other countries, which have decentralized operational responsibilities and resources for the water and sanitation sector to local governments and their organizations. They are especially relevant in the light of the global efforts to meet the new Millennium Development Goals, which the United Nations set in its plenary meeting on 8 September 2000 and at the World Summit on Social Development in Johannesburg in 2003. For water and sanitation, these are to halve, by 2015, the proportion of people who have no access to safe drinking water and/or basic sanitation.

A LANDSCAPE OF MODELS

In the previous sections of the book, a landscape of models, the major findings and conclusions on current experiences in India were presented and discussed. This is now followed by an agenda of research that can support the large-scale application of managed water supply and sanitation by rural communities and the supporting organizations at above-community levels. In the operationalization of the new sector-related policies and programmes, the state governments and their institutions played a crucial role, but other models to establish based services also exist. The central government sets national policies for the water sector and finances national programmes. However, it can only encourage implementation as each state sets its own water policies and implements its own programmes (Barot, Ch. 6). In the process, several institutional settings for implementation have evolved on the ground.

Autonomous community initiatives: Cases in which individual communities have effectively improved their water or sanitation conditions on their own initiatives have always existed. The new legislation has increased opportunities for doing so. In Kerala and Madhya Pradesh, for example, communities have effectively implemented their own water and (school) sanitation projects, using their own resources and accessing additional funds under a government programme or a programme for bilateral cooperation (Sankar, Ch. 3; Kumar, Ch. 7).

Gender needs and strategies, with women uniting to overcome resistance among the local elites and with the government bureaucracy, were important for the success of these projects (Kumar, Ch. 7). Presumably, these projects are not cleared by any line department except for the one under which they are funded.

State experiments with bilateral funds: In Andhra Pradesh, Gujarat, Kerala and Uttar Pradesh, the state water agencies have implemented water supply projects with community participation and management under bilateral financing. The degree of control decentralized to communities in these projects has been limited; planning and management remained in the hands of the water utilities. The limited devolution happened under pressure from the donor and did not change implementation modes of the agencies in their other projects (Sijbesma, Ch. 10). After two decades of financing these capital-intensive agency-driven projects, the Netherlands therefore funded village-managed water pilot projects in one district of each state except in the case of Uttar Pradesh, with some promising results.

State projects parallel to the existing state and local government structure: In Uttar Pradesh, the state government used a loan from the World Bank to contract out implementation to a separate project organization. These contracted NGOs and private consultants help rural communities set up water and sanitation committees and plan, implement and manage local water supplies and related interventions. Local governments were not formally involved. In contrast, the parallel model in Gujarat links with the existing government structure. WASMO is a registered society financed with bilateral funds. It assists Panchayat institutions to plan and manage water within the community boundaries. The state water board manages the outside parts of the water schemes and supports the work technically (Reddy, Ch. 5).

Community projects under decentralized local government (district) programmes: The Sector Reform pilot project enabled villages in 63 districts to access central government funds to plan and implement their own water and sanitation projects. Newly formed District Agencies cleared technical proposals and allocated funds and NGOs to support community organization and planning (Kumar, Ch. 7).

Counter-reacting to the loss of control over funding and implementation support, state water agencies have also taken up this moderating role in spite of their lack of social expertise and experience with small-scale water supply technologies and community-managed services (Reddy, Ch. 5; Kumar, Ch. 7; Shordt, Ch. 9).

Community projects under NGO programmes: Alongside rural water programmes of state governments, NGOs such as Utthan have assisted rural communities to plan and undertake their own water supply improvements. Empowering women and poor people suffering from water scarcity to implement locally sustainable water technologies became the main strategy for drought-prone districts in Gujarat (Barot, Ch. 6).

Public-private partnerships: In a number of communities , the formal and informal private sector supplies drinking water to supplement or replace poorly functioning public services. Either the consumers have formed their own society which built and runs a private water supply (Sankar, Ch. 3) or private entrepreneurs responded to local demand with the silent consent of the municipality (Reddy and Dev, Ch. 4; James and Moriarty, Ch. 10). Furthermore, contractors have assisted communities to construct water supplies under the Sector Reform Project (Kumar, Ch. 7).

HOW BEAUTIFUL IS SMALL FOR THE BIG?

In implementation, there have been a number of positive experiences for all these models. Community water supplies built under bilateral or government funding with participation from men and women in local planning have provided better access for all, including the poor households, than has been the case in projects with no participatory planning. Local planning and management have also contributed to better service performance and greater community self-reliance for drinking water (Barot, Ch. 6; Kumar, Ch. 7; Sijbesma, Ch. 8). Within three years, the output of demand-based panchayat-managed sanitation in Kerala was three times higher than in the supply-driven state programme. The latrines are also generally used, against only 40 per cent of Maharashtra's 1.4 million latrines built under a supply-driven programme (Sankar, Ch. 3).

Privately managed small-scale community water supplies are also more effective and efficient as reported in the case studies of Sankar (Ch. 3), Reddy and Dev (Ch. 4) and James and Moriarty (Ch. 10). Adjustment of connection costs to their income patterns made joining the schemes more affordable for the poor (Sankar, Box 3.2).

At the same time, implementation of locally managed water supply and sanitation has been limited, slow and far from ideal. The response of state bureaucracies to the scaling up of community-planned and managed services has been disappointing (Reddy, Ch. 5). Lessons gained in experiments under bilateral and multilateral cooperation are reflected in policy and programmes at national level, but the states have been reluctant to mainstream them in their own policies and programmes.

Under the new national policy, all implementation shifted to local government (panchayat) institutions. However, the pilot project in 63 districts did not go according to plan. Opposition came particularly from the state water supply and sanitation agencies, which saw their fund flow and control in the sector get reduced and the role of NGOs being increased. Their lobby resulted in a shift in policy in November 2002. A new, nationwide programme for community-planned and -managed rural water supply, Swajaldhara, was set up alongside the pilot. Its guidelines de-emphasize software, capacity development, joint planning, and departmental collaboration (Shordt, Ch. 9). Subsequently, the Ministry of Rural Development ended the pilot because of insufficient support and poor results. Many of the released funds were either not used or misappropriated (*The Hindu*, 3 May 2003). One half-year later, the national policy was again changed, reverting to lines quite similar to the pre-November 2002 policy.

In the revamped programme, state water agencies retrieved their key position in rural water supply and sanitation. The existing agencies for rural drinking water supply—which until then had implemented supply-driven, non-participatory projects—remained the implementers (Swajaldhara guidelines, http://ddws.nic.in/DDWS_Swajal.htm, 22 April 2003). Communities can only work with NGOs or any other support organization when these are cleared and contracted by the state water agencies or the district committees of which they are a member. A national project for building organizational and human capacity ended prematurely (Shordt, Ch. 9).

This 'tied aid' (the 90 per cent government-paid Swajaldhara is the only large programme for community management and communities can only work with government engineers and government-approved NGOs) comes with delays. The bureaucracy decides, but does not have to meet process deadlines and is not accountable for performance as in Swajal. This has led to technical and procedural delays in making contracts and clearing community proposals. Contracting NGOs has sometimes taken two years. There are also too few NGOs with substantial experience in water and sanitation for this large programme. A combination of no rules (for preparing projects) and too much bureaucracy, so that community members cannot do their own acquisition and submission of tenders at competitive prices, is another impediment (Reddy, Ch. 5; Kumar, Ch. 7).

Some communities have the leadership, contacts and expertise that enable them to undertake improvements autonomously such as the ones reported by Sankar (Ch. 3) and Kumar (Ch. 7). However, these cases have been few and far between.

Stimulating NGO programmes is another model. Many of them (but not all) have faith in village capacities and skills to help communities undertake their own projects with gender and social equity. The Swajal project has shown that NGOs which are shortlisted for their social experience and managerial capacities, had no problems in engaging engineers for helping local women and men make informed technology choices and take up technical tasks. However, without government financing of capital costs (90 per cent under Swajaldhara), the scope of work of NGOs in the rural water sector is limited. In Gujarat, for example, Utthan could assist 108 villages in four districts and took up 28 watershed development projects (Barot, Ch. 6). Officially, Gujarat has only 1,532 un-served or partially served communities, so in that case 108 would be substantial. However, the statistics leave out many communities with perennial water shortage (Reddy, Ch. 5).

In its current forms, PPPs have been partial solutions. Cases of partnerships with the formal and informal sectors have been few and far between and have pros and cons. The experiences reported by Sankar (Ch. 3), Reddy and Dev (Ch. 4) and James and Moriarty (Ch. 10) show that piped water supply operated by private entrepreneurs or by a user association provided a better service to the middle and upper classes, but excluded the poor. In the Sector Reform Project, private contractors have sometimes made the designs and paid the 10 per cent community contributions for interested communities. The contractors recovered these costs and increased their own profits by designing costlier schemes and including speed charges (Kumar, Ch. 7). Overall, experiences with small enterprises reported in this book have been more positive than with larger companies and financing organizations (Satyanarayana, Ch. 11).

For rural sanitation, the campaign with small private sector involvement has potential, but there are concerns about the preservation of the quality of the process and results. A full strategy consists of helping express hidden demands (especially among women and middle class) and creating new demands (among men and the poor), meeting these demands through the local private sector and the sanitation shops of NGOs, CBOs and enterprising households, and promoting and monitoring use and hygiene by all. The campaign is being scaled up rapidly, covering already over 330 districts by the end of 2003. There are concerns that its quantitative targets will result merely in the construction of toilets, at the expense of process quality and the use of the facilities. Another concern is the position of hygiene promotion. It is now a part of Information, Education and Communication (IEC), which tends to be dominated by building awareness of sanitation options rather than promoting and evaluating latrine use and hygiene (UNICEF, 2003).

CONCLUSIONS: POLITICAL AND INSTITUTIONAL CHANGE

The challenges in India to meet the Millennium Development Goals are political and institutional, rather than purely financial or technical. Politically, there is the challenge that political parties at the state and national level embrace local government reforms not just in words, but also in deeds. Major bottlenecks for the new policy and programme to meet the Millennium Development Goals for (sustained) access (and use) in the water sector are: the reluctance of the states to transfer funds, functionaries and functions as well as authority to panchayats and no willingness to build capacities at the lowest levels—the elected governments, the water and sanitation committees and the user assemblies. For improvements in the water and sanitation sector, rural communities do not depend, however, on the delegation of state funds alone. Swajaldhara provides national funds which in principle allow them to improve their rural water supply and sanitation to a level which they can and will maintain and use.

Local capacities for panchayat-managed water supply and sanitation need strengthening, but local resources for doing so are present. Scoping has shown that in general districts had both capacity building resources and the political will to use them. It needed facilitators to assist in bringing stakeholders together and help them match obstacles to resources to enable them to prepare district capacity development plans. However, the rapid changes in the programme have seriously slowed down the district scoping activity and the development of scoping capacities in the programme.

An institutional problem is that communities cannot fulfill the necessary functions without having access to the necessary skills and functionaries. The functionaries that dominate implementation have no experience with participatory planning and management of rural water supplies, no expertise on and experience with gender and poverty approaches, and have not worked as partners with NGOs that do have the required experience and skills. State water supply agencies which are steeped in traditional centralized, supply-driven approaches have insisted that they remain the lead agency for Swajaldhara. Some district authorities and political parties have also resented the shift of power and have been reluctant to trust local development capacities and delegate funds and control. Scoping has helped districts to pinpoint and address local bottlenecks with local resources. It has not transformed the supporting institutions.

The success of Swajaldhara is further threatened by, and constitutes a threat to, the adequate management of water resources in India. The threat to the programme comes from the ongoing process of depletion and contamination of freshwater resources summarized at the start of this chapter. When the lowering of freshwater quality and quantity goes on and resource competition from agriculture, cities and industries increases, many rural communities will again run out of safe drinking water. Swajaldhara itself may well contribute to inter-sector competition when increasing living standards raise demands for private house connections in water-scarce areas without accompanying water demand management. It may also contribute to the contamination of shallow water tables from an increasing number of soak pit latrines. In both situations the poor are likely to be most affected as they have no storage reservoirs and rely on public hand pumps, taps and open water sources. Moreover, as few rural communities can treat drinking water and/or transport it over large distances, they will yet come to depend on centrally managed, large water schemes that are costly to install and maintain.

To meet new demands for water for drinking, sanitation and hygiene, and domestic economic use in a short time and at politically acceptable tariffs will be difficult for government and the private sector. Instead of improving, it is possible that the rural water and sanitation situation will deteriorate if the water resources aspects of Swajaldhara are not addressed.

While the decentralization policy has been adopted at the national level, individual states move at different speeds in the devolution of the three Fs—Funds, Functions and Functionaries. At the state level, support for decentralization and community management is in particular insufficient for the water sector. This is partly due to a lack of common definitions and understanding. This could be addressed through dialogue on the basis of carefully developed information material and information campaigns designed to reach each group through the appropriate channels and not with government messages, but with information tailored to their demands.

The implementation does not change the fact that decentralization and community management have been imposed from the top. The state water agencies are not keen to support community management. Their staff has little interest in low-cost sanitation and many feel that the new rural water supply policy threatens their current positions. The policy is further undermined by substantial groups which place their faith in mega-projects such as the Narmada Project and the plan to interconnect Indian rivers. While large-scale solutions are unproven, they serve as excuses not to change the existing rural water supply approaches and programmes.

Supporting community-managed water supply and low-cost sanitation programmes requires that these approaches change and are fed by a different knowledge, attitudes and skills mix. Few engineers in state water agencies could develop this mix during their education and work. At the same time, they are reluctant to hand over support roles to other agencies.

The review has shown that there are also other ways of implementing decentralized management of water supply and sanitation. Consequently, there is a need to test different models for decentralized water supply and sanitation with different options of institutional support.

One option is the mobilization of volunteers among young engineers in engineering departments who want to develop their capabilities for community-managed water supply and low-cost sanitation. Institutionally, they could form a special unit or units within the water agencies or, if salary levels allow, be attached to the districts along with social specialists or work in partnerships with social specialists in NGOs. In either case, the Swajaldhara programme would need to provide them with opportunities to develop their capabilities and build up an alternative career in community engineering.

The task of these specialized, multidisciplinary units would be to develop, test and document district and state strategies for implementing community management of rural water supplies and household latrine programmes. In doing so they would be asked to pay specific attention to emerging key issues. Technically, they would assist communities with combinations of rehabilitation, upgrading and new construction to achieve a reliable, equitable and holistic system of community water supply for drinking, cooking, hygiene and basic productivity within households, along with improved sanitation. Technology options and service levels should be acceptable and manageable for different types of communities and households. Socially, the teams would devise, test and document ways to reach the poor and ensure that women and poor women have equal shares in decisions and benefits. Financially, they would help communities to achieve equitable sharing of partial community financing of capital costs and full financing of operation and maintenance cost. The financing systems would be locally specific and planned, and include accountability to the users, including women and poor households. Environmentally, they would help communities to develop adequate management of water and waste disposal throughout local catchment areas with representation of all stakeholder groups according to sex, class and water uses. Institutionally, the aim would be to achieve effective and equitable management of services with accountability for performance including to the poor and women.

Letting communities choose their own supporting and implementing agencies, be they from government, NGOs or the private sector is another option. Government financing of the investment costs would then include compensation for the organizations that assist communities in making the proposal and designs.

Government financing for NGO programmes for community-managed water supply and sanitation would be another model. NGO financing could be tried alongside existing modalities. The strength of such an approach would be the social expertise and holistic water resources and catchment approaches which are missing in state water agencies.

The participation process itself cannot be time bound. Some communities need more time to come to a decision than others and community women and men must combine their work as volunteers on water and sanitation with their regular tasks. Swajaldhara can, however, reward timely action by paid workers at above-community levels.

CONTRIBUTIONS FROM APPLIED RESEARCH

Gaining support, trying new institutional support models, and testing and documenting field approaches are crucial for the success of Swajaldhara and for learning more about the effects of decentralization. Applied research, in particular the identification and analysis of good practices and action research for hands-on analysis and improvement of current approaches and evaluation of effects, can play a useful role. Since change has to come from within, the type of research will be participatory. The following topics emerged from the papers and the group discussions during the seminar:

Learning from pilot experiences: The national Swajaldhara Programme is being implemented without systematically learning from and critical documentation of the projects on which it is based. It is, therefore, not known how effective and efficient these projects have been in creating sustained and equitable services, and with which support approaches and costs for investments and support.

Institutional and political leadership: Another research subject is whether in any of the pilot areas, institutions and leaders at the block, district and state level have modified their approaches to become effective supporters of the sector reforms and if so, for which reasons. Thus, important insights can be gained into how institutional and leadership reforms come about which make it possible to scale up community-managed water services and sanitation programmes under various forms of lowest level management.

Best practices: A further area for study is to identify best practices regarding, among others, who participates in what and to what effect, to whom institutions account and for what, how services are financed and costs covered, how autonomous institutions can make their services efficient and effective, and which forms of adaptive management and partnerships between actors (panchayat institutions, district authorities, water utilities, civic groups and users) have led to a more effective and equitable supply of water, including to the poor and marginal groups.

Political leadership: Research questions identified with regard to political leadership were the use of more appropriate technologies and service level mixes; the adoption of more realistic water tariffs with equity for the poor; acceptance of a greater autonomy for utilities and communities to install and manage services that they can sustain and that can serve, and continue to serve all without unduly advantaging certain groups; access for the poor and women to decision making, training and entrepreneurship; and appreciation of the importance of sanitation and willingness to abandon subsidies and invest in creating and meeting demands.

Demand management and supply efficiency: Very few systematic and scientific studies on demand management are available to guide policies. A first step to their execution and the use of findings is that policy makers become convinced of the usefulness of such research. Good demand studies will investigate who—including the poor and women—has which kind of demands and collect valid, locally specific statistics for the various uses. Action research is possible to test demand management through pricing and metering. Where meters are not possible, alternative measures to reduce consumption and link prices to amounts of water consumed can be tested such as a higher tariff based on agreed socio-economic indicators (households with a higher socio-economic status consume more water than households with a lower status). Increased awareness and new norms to reduce water wastage and the creation of a demand for, and supply of, water saving devices can also reduce the consumption of drinking water. Affordable and effective methods have also be developed to raise the awareness of water scarcity and the range of countervailing practices and measures.

Technical, social and managerial measures for unaccounted for water and different technologies and designs can be tested to increase the efficiency of supply, including a more holistic use of different water systems in one community or area. Benchmarking, or comparing performance of different utilities or communities on common standards and with the same measurement methods, can help create more transparency and accountability for results against costs, including for services to the poor. In the area of water resources, research is needed to determine the effects of bans on groundwater withdrawal and impacts on water availability and access. Social research can help make consumer groups more aware of groundwater data and use these to protect drinking water supply and counteract over-exploitation for private profit. Much can be gained by concerted action from all water-related sectors for better water management and supply efficiency, involving actors at every level, to begin from within households. Experiments with such concerted action can be given a high research priority.

Research on the processes and impacts of sector reforms in India are of national and global importance. National, because the sector reform is the greatest change since the adoption of the Accelerated Rural Water Supply and Minimum Needs Programmes in India in the 1970s, programmes which have brought access to improved facilities, but not yet sustained and for all. Internationally, because progress in achieving access to *and* sustained and year-round use of safe water and sanitation by all in the country with the second largest population in the world will have substantial impact on global conditions and sets a reference point for others.

Seeing the importance of the sector, the scope of the reform programme and the relevance of applied research to addresses the key bottlenecks in realizing the national water and sanitation policies, it is surprising that India has not yet led to a specific research programme or programmes on domestic water supply and sanitation. It is hoped that the initiative of bringing together economic and social researchers to report on innovative experiences and the identification of an agenda for further research will contribute to the emergence of such a programme.

List of Contributors

Meine Pieter van Dijk, Ph.D., Economist
Professor of Water Services Management
UNESCO IHE Institute for Water Education
P.O. Box 3015, 2601 DA Delft, The Netherlands
T + 31-152151779
F + 31-10-4089153
E m.vandijk@unesco-ihe.org

Ulaganathan Sankar, Ph.D., Economist
Honorary Professor
Madras School of Economics
Gandhi Mandapam Road, Chennai 600 025
T + 91-44-235 2157
F + 91-44-235 4847
E msepu@md3.vsnl.net.in , sankar_u75@hotmail.com

V. Ratna Reddy, Ph.D., Economist
Professor
Centre for Economic and Social Studies
N.O. Campus, Begumpet, Hyderabad 500 016, India
T + 91 40 23402789
F + 91 40 23406808
E vratnareddy@cess.ac.in

S. Mahendra Dev, Ph.D., Economist
Professor and Director
Centre for Economic and Social Studies
N.O. Campus, Begumpet, Hyderabad 500 016, India
T + 91 40 23402789
F + 91 40 23406808
E smahendradev@cess.ac.in

J.S. Burjia, I.A.S.
Joint Secretary
Government of India, Ministry of Water Resources
Shram Shakti Bhawan
New Delhi 110 001
T + 91-11-2371 0343
E jsburjia@nic.in

Christine Sijbesma, Ph.D., Sociologist
Senior Programme Officer
IRC International Water and Sanitation Centre
P.O. Box 2869, 2601 CW Delft, The Netherlands
T +31 15 2192939 (R) +31 73 5994234
F +31 15 2190955
E christinevanwijk@gmail.com

K. Prathap Reddy, Ph.D.
Professor and Director,
Institute of Rural Management Anand (IRMA)
Post Box 60, Anand - 388 001, Gujarat, India
T +91-02692-261230; (R) +91-02692-261880/261995
F +91-02692-260188
E kpr@fac.irm.ernet.in

Nafisa Barot, Ms.
Executive Trustee
Utthan – Development Action Planning Team
36, Chitrakut Twins, Nehru Park, Vastrapur
Ahmedabad - 380015, Gujarat, India
T + 91 079 6751023; 6762875; 6732926
F + 91 079 6750935; 6763624
E Utthan@icenet.net , nafisa@icenet.net

Yogesh Kumar
Director
Samarth (NGO)
Bhopal, Madya Pradesh
samarth@bom6.vsnl.net.in

A.J. James
Environmental & Natural Resource Economist
609B Hamilton Court
DLF City Phase IV
Gurgaon 122 002, India
T +91- 124 (95124 from Delhi) 505 1338 M 981011 3698
E ajjames@vsnl.net

Patrick Moriarty, Ph.D.
Head - Knowledge Development and Advocacy
IRC International Water and Sanitation Centre
P.O. Box 2869, 2601 CW Delft, The Netherlands
T +31 15 2192939 (R) +31 73 5994234
F +31 15 2190955
E moriarty@irc.nl

Kathleen Shordt, BSc, M.Ed.
IRC International Water and Sanitation Centre
P.O. Box 2869, 2601 CW Delft, The Netherlands
T +31 15 2192939 (R) +31 73 5994234
F +31 15 2190955
E shordt@irc.nl

V. Satyanarayna
Senior Infrastructure Finance Advisor
Financial Institutions Reform and Expansion (FIRE) Project
E- 3/4 Vasant Vihar, New Delhi 110 057 India
T +91-11-2614 9836/ 2614 3551/ 2615 1081-3, ext 16
F +91-11-2614 1420
E satya@indo-usfired.com

Index